DR. **IKKAKU OCHI** COLLECTION

WITH CONTRIBUTIONS / MIT BEITRÄGEN VON

ANNA VON SENGER **SUMIO ISHIDA AKIMITSU NARUYAMA**

SCALO

SUMIO ISHIDA

Born in 1948 in the prefecture of Okayama, Japan. He graduated from the medical faculty of the University of Okayama in 1973. Ishida is a physician, doctor of medicine and a professor at the University of Niimi, Okayama (medical faculty), and Hiroshima (history of medicine). He is also the director of the *Japan Society of Medical History*.

Geboren 1948 in der Präfektur Okayama, Japan. 1973 schloß er sein Studium an der medizinischen Fakultät der Universität Okayama ab. Ishida ist praktizierender Arzt, Doktor der Medizin und Professor an den Universitäten Niimi, Okayama (medizinische Fakultät) und Hiroshima (Geschichte der Medizin). Zudem ist er Vorstand der *Japan Society of Medical History*.

AKIMITSU NARUYAMA

Born in 1966 in Tokyo, Japan. In his childhood he was trained in traditional Japanese music like koto. Later he started to collect surrealist photographs and drawings. In 1997 he opened Gallery Naruyama in the Kudan neighborhood in Tokyo. His personal collections as well as his exhibitions, which reflect a sad and timeless beauty, attract people from all over the world.

Geboren 1966 in Tokio, Japan. Bereits in seiner Kindheit wurde er in traditioneller japanischer Musik, zum Beispiel Koto, unterrichtet. Später begann Naruyama, surrealistische Fotografien und Zeichnungen zu sammeln. 1997 eröffnete er die Galerie Naruyama im Tokioter Viertel Kudan. Seine persönlichen Sammlungen und seine Ausstellungen, die eine traurige und zeitlose Schönheit ausstrahlen, ziehen Menschen aus der ganzen Welt in ihren Bann.

ANNA VON SENGER

Born in 1967, the daughter of a Swiss father and a Japanese mother, she spent her childhood in Tokyo. She lives and works as a freelance journalist in Zurich and is the mother of two children.

1967 als Tochter eines Schweizers und einer Japanerin geboren, verbrachte Anna von Senger ihre Kindheit in Tokio. Sie lebt als freiberufliche Journalistin in Zürich und ist Mutter zweier Kinder.

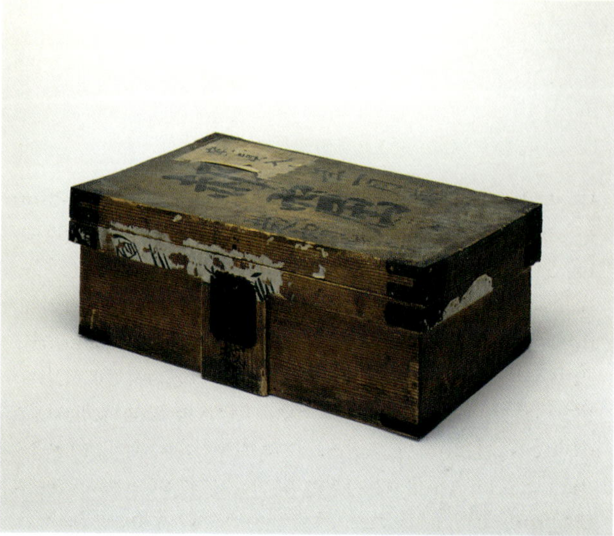

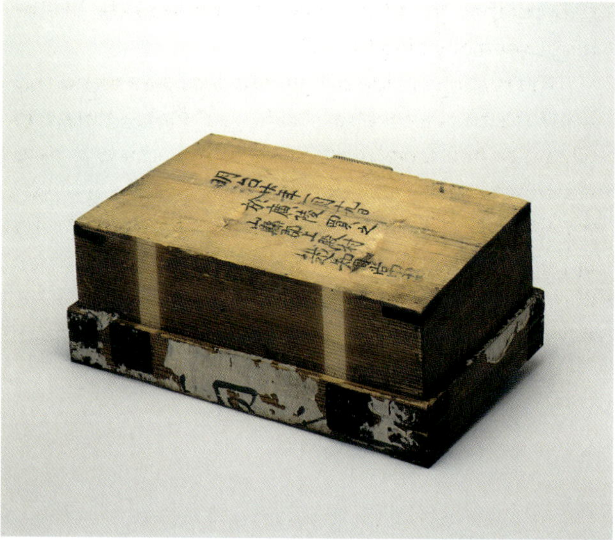

THE COLLECTION OF DR. IKKAKU OCHI

MEDICAL PHOTOGRAPHY FROM JAPAN AROUND 1900

IN JAPANESE FAIRYTALES and legends we often encounter boxes. They are farewell presents the protagonist receives upon leaving another world. The protagonist must not open the box, yet this very prohibition forces him to do so. Boxes are full of secrets. And it is in human nature to want to reveal them. This type of secret started my discovery of this collection of medical photographs. One day, the art collector Akimitsu Naruyama, a long-time friend of mine, called me from Tokyo. "I got a box with more than 300 incredible photographs," he told me. "They are medical photographs from the Meiji era (1868–1911). You've never seen anything like it."

The box was made of light princess-tree wood and was the size of a shoebox. "Kakugan" (kaku=a place in China, gan=a cave) and an illegible name and date were written in Kanji on its stained lid. On its back was the name and the date of an earlier owner. In the upper right corner, someone had pasted a thin piece of rice paper with the note "Content: photographs." A quick glance inside explained Naruyama's excitement:

it contained hundreds of photographs of people with congenital or pathological deformations. Even to a medical amateur it was immediately obvious that these were astonishing historical documents since modern medicine entirely, or at least partially, prevents these deformations from developing. To some, these photographs might go too far. Nevertheless, it was impossible to ignore the beauty of some of these images. They are not merely documents of disease. Rather, they are sensitive portraits of humans enduring their ordeals with a stoic, or even dignified, attitude. They tell us about the deformations afflicting the young, adult, and aging, the real and the idealized human body. They tell us about the melancholia in between the ideal and the real.

There were altogether 365 photographs in the box—five on glass plates, the rest were albumin prints on cardboard. There were eye, skin, and venereal diseases, moreover they also showed tumors and congenital deformations. 150 photographs were numbered on the back, complemented by the name of the photographer's studio and the name of the disease. Hence, you could assume that it was a complete set. Besides this set, the box contained photographs by the medical faculty of the University of Kyoto (Daisan-Kotochugakko) in Okayama (the prefecture of Okayama is in the south of Japan, bordering on Hiroshima to the west), some portraits and class photographs. These images were signed on the back by a certain Ikkaku Ochi with his name and address. Ochi was born on February 15 (or June 12), 1875, in Uedono-mura in Sanken-gun in the prefecture of Hiroshima. In 1895, he graduated from the medical faculty of the University of Kyoto in Okayama, together with 62 other students. In 1896, he joined the Japanese army as medical officer until his honorable discharge in 1917. Among others, he served on the frontlines of the Japanese-Russian war (1904–1905). In 1918, he opened a practice for internal medicine in the city of Hiroshima where he died on January 21, 1930. It is no longer possible to determine how and where he acquired the photographs. Most likely they are educational material he obtained during his studies at the University of Kyoto. Astonishingly, they even survived the nuclear attack on Hiroshima.

The starting point of the search for the photographer was the name of the photo studio printed on the back, *Ôta Shashinkan* (shashinkan=photo studio) and its address. The studio was located in the Nishi-Sange neighborhood in the city of Okayama, directly opposite the council house. It was also called *Ôta Rakusui-ken*, according to an ad in the local directory of small businesses and industry. Thanks to one of his descendants who conducts research on his ancestors on the internet, we could determine the name of the photographer and studio owner at the time: Tsutomu Ôta.

In 1868, he was born the third son of physician Yoan Moriya in Kurashiki, Okayama. His father was well-known for his efforts in the fight against the smallpox virus. Tsutomu's older brother Hoichiro continued the family tradition and became a medical officer. As was custom when a family lacked male descendants, he took on the name of his wife's family, Ôta. The Ôta family (among them were a few physicians, too) had been civil servants for generations, but increasingly lost their power and wealth during the Meiji restoration. To pay off debts Tsutomu had to sell the family's house in the village of Nishi-Hanajiri in Okayama and moved with his family to the city of Okayama. He first worked as a security guard at a school which turned out to be a fortunate coincidence for a student asked him to guard his camera, then still rare and expensive, during classes. Tsutomu Ôta taught himself how to use the camera and soon opened up his own photo studio, *Ôta Rakusui-ken*.

Most likely Tsutomu was soon commissioned to photograph patients with rare symptoms of diseases. In 1890, a photograph by Tsutomu was already published in the medical journal *Geibi Iji*. He was only 22-years old at the time. Most likely it was a commission by the authors of these studies who all taught at the medical faculty and worked at the affiliated hospital of the prefecture of Okayama where they treated these patients. The hospital was only half a mile away from Tsutomu's studio. In addition it was probably helpful that his brother Hoichiro had studied at the same faculty and hence had contacts at the hospital. The photographs probably were archival documents of rare diseases. Looking through old issues of *Geibi Iji* in the library of the medical faculty at the University of Okayama, we found five of the patients photographed by Ôta. Since photographs were not printed in large editions back then, Tsutomu Ôta's photographs were copied as copperplate engravings, which were then used as illustrations in *Geibi Iji*.

For instance the young woman with bilateral mammahyperplasia (oversized breasts) on whom the physician Genshi Seo reported the following in the issue of May 31, 1890: the girl whose last name was Ono had been rather weak since birth. In 1888, when she was 16-years old, she had her first period and noticed at the same time that her breasts were starting to grow. After 12 months, they developed to a "normal" size, yet the quantity of menstrual blood decreased every month. Her breasts kept growing while she simultaneously lost weight. When she weighed no more than 81 pounds and could no longer carry the weight of her breasts, the doctors started to fear for her life. At the urgent request of the young woman, they decided to amputate both breasts. The operation was performed on December 17, 1889. The right breast weighed 4.8 pounds, whereas the left breast weighed 4.6 pounds, adding up to 1/9 of her entire weight. "No wonder, Miss Ono kept losing weight for 1/9 of her diet went right into this parasitic organ." Three weeks later, Miss Ono left the hospital in good health, weighing more than 100 pounds. (p. 91/92)

Or the 26-year old man with a dilation of the stomach (gastrectasia) whose "extraordinarily extreme dimensions" made Dr. Shinichi Kodama of the hospital of the prefecture Okayama almost gush. Mr. Uemori came to the hospital on May 27, 1895, when he was no longer able to continue his work as rice thresher. Since puberty he suffered from chronic constipation. With 17 he was diagnosed with a stomach disease. It was treated and cured in 1892 at the prefecture hospital. Two years later, however, his stomach started to swell. "The maximum circumference of his stomach was one yard when he visited the hospital. When the patient was lying on his back, you could clearly make out a writhing movement in the stomach area. It intensified when you touched it with your hand, something cold, or an electric current. Through the stethoscope you could hear a low throbbing, and the stomach felt like a gigantic inflatable cushion," the doctor continued. "It is unusual that despite these symptoms Mr. Uemori has more or less healthy digestion and goes to stool once a day." When the stomach was examined more closely, it turned out that the amount of pepsin (a ferment of the stomach fluids that splits proteins) was normal. Dr. Kodama suspected that the cause for the disease was a mechanical malfunction of the pylorus, the connection between the stomach and the duodenum. (p. 85)

In 1897, a physician named Tachisaburo Sarai reported a case of tetanus with grave effects. The 24-year old man had fallen ill with tetanus at the age of 9 and had not been able to move his lower jaw ever since. He could only eat mashed food through an opening where his teeth had fallen out. Full of compassion, Dr. Sarai wrote, "He has never eaten a *manju* (Japanese shortbread cookie), he only knows the juice of mandarins, and he eats noodles by 'chewing' them with his lips and his tongue." The patient had a hard time articulating, but you could more or less understand what he said. On December 24, 1896, the joint of the right lower jaw was cut through. The patient got off lightly: he had to be reanimated because of a cyanosis. Two days later, his articulation had clearly improved, and on December 30 he already ate three bowls of rice. On January 20 of the following year the same operation was performed on the left side. Once again, there were some complications. On April 7, the doctor noted the right half of his face was more or less normal. (p. 153)

These are only three case histories—we only know the faces of the other patients and the aura surrounding them. But each of them has a story to tell of a life changed by illness, with passing or lasting effects.

Anna von Senger

OFT SPIELEN IN JAPANISCHEN Sagen und Märchen Schachteln eine Rolle. Es sind Geschenke zum Abschied aus einer anderen Welt, die nicht geöffnet werden dürfen, was wiederum die Protagonisten zwingt, genau dies zu tun. Schachteln sind somit voller Geheimnisse. Und es liegt in der menschlichen Natur, diese lüften zu wollen. Ein solches Geheimnis stand auch am Anfang der Entdeckung dieser Sammlung von Medizinfotografien. Eines Tages rief mich mein langjähriger Freund, der Kunstsammler Akimitsu Naruyama, aus Tokio an: »Ich bin im Besitz einer Schachtel mit mehr als 300 unglaublichen Fotografien«, teilte er mir mit. »Es sind medizinische Fotos aus der Meiji-Ära (1868–1911). So etwas hast du noch nie gesehen.«

Die Schachtel war aus leichtem Kaiserbaumholz und hatte etwa die Größe einer Schuhschachtel. Auf dem verschmutzten Deckel stand in großen Kanji-Schriftzeichen »kakugan« (*kaku*=eine Ortschaft in China, *gan*=Höhle), dazu unleserlich ein Datum und ein Name. Auf der Rückseite stand der Name eines früheren Nutzers und ein Datum, und oben rechts klebte auf dünnem Reispapier geschrieben der Hinweis »Inhalt: Fotografien«. Der Blick ins Innere erklärte Naruyamas Aufregung: Hunderte Fotos von Menschen mit angeborenen und krankheitsbedingten Deformationen kamen zum Vorschein. Selbst einem medizinischen Laien mußte augenblicklich klar werden, welch interessante Zeitdokumente er in seinen Händen hielt – denn die abgebildeten Symptome oder Mißbildungen entwickeln sich heute dank der modernen Medizin nicht mehr oder nicht so weit. Für manche Augen mögen sie auch zu weit gehen. Trotzdem war die Schönheit einiger Bilder nicht zu übersehen. Sie dokumentieren nicht nur Krankheiten, sondern sind oft auch einfühlsame Porträts von Menschen, die ihre Leiden stoisch oder gar mit Würde zu ertragen scheinen. Und sie erzählen von den Deformationen, denen der junge, der erwachsene und der alternde, denen der reale und der idealisierte menschliche Körper ausgesetzt ist. Sie erzählen von der Melancholie zwischen Ideal und Realität.

Insgesamt befanden sich 356 Fotografien in der Schachtel: fünf auf Glasplatten, die restlichen in Albumin-Abzügen auf Karton. Es handelte sich um Augen-, Haut- und Geschlechtskrankheiten, aber auch Tumore und angeborene Mißbildungen. 150 Exemplare waren auf der Rückseite durchnumeriert und mit dem Namen des Fotostudios und der jeweiligen Krankheit bedruckt.

Es mußte sich also um ein vollständiges Set handeln. Zu diesen medizinischen Fotografien gesellten sich Aufnahmen vom Institut der medizinischen Fakultät der Universität Kyoto (Daisan-Kotochugakko) in Okayama (die Präfektur Okayama befindet sich im Süden Japans und grenzt im Westen an Hiroshima), sowie einige Porträts und Klassenfotos. Auf der Rückseite dieser Bilder unterschrieb mit seiner Adresse ein Mann namens Ikkaku Ochi. Ikkaku Ochi wurde am 15. Februar (oder 12. Juni) 1875 in Uedono-mura in Sanken-gun in der Präfektur Hiroshima geboren. 1895 absolviert er mit weiteren 62 Studenten die medizinische Fakultät der Universität Kyoto in Okayama. 1896 tritt er als Militärarzt in die japanische Armee ein, bis er sie 1917 verläßt. Unter anderem ist er im Japanisch-Russischen Krieg (1904/1905) an der Front tätig. 1918 eröffnet Ochi eine Praxis für innere Medizin in der Stadt Hiroshima. Dort stirbt er am 21. Januar 1930. Wie er zu den Fotografien kam, kann heute nicht mehr geklärt werden. Höchstwahrscheinlich erhielt er sie zu Studienzwecken von der Universität. Erstaunlich ist, daß sie den Atombombenangriff auf Hiroshima heil überstanden haben.

Als Anhaltspunkt auf der Suche nach dem Fotografen dienten der Name des Fotostudios »Ôta Shashinkan« (*shashinkan*=Fotostudio), und dessen Adresse, die auf die Fotokarten gedruckt waren. Das Studio befand sich im Nishi-Sange-Bezirk in der Stadt Okayama, gegenüber dem Rathaus. Wie ein Inserat im lokalen Industrie- und Gewerbeanzeiger dieser Zeit zeigt, nannte es sich auch »Ôta Rakusui-ken«. Dank einem Nachkommen, der Ahnenforschung auf dem Internet betreibt, konnte der Name des damaligen Studiobesitzers und Fotografen ausfindig gemacht werden: Tsutomu Ôta.

Er wurde 1868 als dritter Sohn des Arztes Yoan Moriya in Kurashiki, Okayama, geboren. Sein Vater wurde bekannt durch sein Engagement im Kampf gegen Pockenviren. Tsutomus großer Bruder Hoichiro führte als Erstgeborener die Familientradition fort und wurde Militärarzt. Tsutomu heiratete sich aber in die Familie seiner Frau ein und nahm deren Namen, Ôta, an – wie in dieser Zeit üblich, wenn Mangel an männlichen Nachkommen herrschte. Die Ôtas – eine Familie, die ebenfalls einige Ärzte hervorbrachte – waren seit Generationen Beamte, welche aber durch die Meiji-Restauration immer mehr an Macht und Reichtum verloren. Um Schulden zu bezahlen, mußte Tsutomu den Familiensitz im Dorf Nishi-Hanajiri in Okayama verkaufen und übersiedelte mit seiner Familie in die Stadt Okayama. Dort arbeitete er zunächst als Sicherheitsbeamter an einer Schule, was sich als glückliche Fügung erweisen sollte. Denn ein Schüler übergab dem Sicherheitsmann seinen damals kostbaren Fotoapparat zur Aufbewahrung während der Schulstunden. Tsutomu Ôta erlernte damit autodidaktisch den Umgang mit der Kamera und eröffnete wenig später sein eigenes Fotostudio »Ôta Rakusui-ken«.

Es dürfte nicht viel Zeit vergangen sein, bis Tsutomu den Auftrag erhielt, Patienten mit seltenen Krankheitssymptomen zu fotografieren. Denn 1890 wird erstmals ein von ihm abgelichteter Patient im Fachjournal »Geibi Iji« gezeigt. Er war damals gerade 22 Jahre alt. Vermutlich kam der Auftrag von den Autoren dieser Abhandlungen, die alle an der medizinischen Fakultät lehrten und im angegliederten Präfekturspital Okayama arbeiteten, wo sie diese Patienten behandelten. Das Spital war nur 800m entfernt von Tsutomus Fotostudio. Hilfreich war sicher auch, daß sein Bruder Hoichiro dieselbe medizinische Fakultät absolviert hatte und so in Verbindung mit dem Spital stand. Höchstwahrscheinlich dienten die Fotografien zur archivarischen Dokumentation seltener Krankheitsfälle. Beim Durchblättern verschiedener Ausgaben von »Geibi Iji« in der Bibliothek der heutigen medizinischen Fakultät der Universität Okayama fanden wir insgesamt fünf von Ôta abgelichtete Patienten. Da Fotografien damals noch nicht in großen Auflagen gedruckt werden konnten, bediente man sich Tsutomu Ôtas Fotos als Vorlagen für Kupferstiche, die dann als Illustrationen in »Geibi Iji« abgedruckt wurden.

Die junge Frau mit einer bilateralen Mammahyperplasie (beidseitig stark vergrößerte Brüste) zum Beispiel, über die der Arzt Genshi Seo in der Ausgabe vom 31. Mai 1890 folgendes berichtet: Das Mädchen mit dem Nachnamen Ono, von Geburt an eher schwächlich, hatte 1888 als 16-Jährige zum ersten Mal ihre Tage und bemerkte gleichzeitig, daß ihre Brüste wuchsen. Nach zwölf Monaten entwickelten sich diese zu »normaler« Größe, die Menge des Menstruationsblutes nahm jedoch monatlich ab. Die Brüste wuchsen indessen weiter, gleichzeitig verlor die junge Frau zusehends an Körpergewicht. Als sie nur noch 37 Kilo wog und sie unter dem Gewicht ihrer Brüste nicht mehr gehen konnte, fürchteten die Ärzte um ihr Leben. Nicht zuletzt auf das Drängen der jungen Frau hin, beschloß man, eine Amputation beider Brüste vorzunehmen. Die Operation erfolgte am 17. Dezember 1889. Das Gewicht der rechten Brust betrug 2,2 Kilo, das der linken 2,1 Kilo, ein Neuntel ihres Körpergewichts. »Kein Wunder, verlor Fräulein Ono immer mehr an Gewicht«, schrieb Dr. Seo, »denn ein Neuntel der Nahrung, die sie aufnahm, ging direkt in dieses parasitäre Organ über.« Drei Wochen später konnte Fräulein Ono das Spital in guter Verfassung und mit einem Gewicht von knapp fünfzig Kilo verlassen. (S.91/92)

Oder der 26-jährige Mann mit einer Magendilatation (Gastrektasie), von deren »besonders extremem Ausmaß« Dr. Shinichi Kodama vom Präfekturspital Okayama regelrecht schwärmte: Herr Uemori suchte am 27. Mai 1895 das Spital auf, als er seiner Tätigkeit als Reisdrescher nicht mehr nachgehen konnte. Er litt seit der Pubertät an chronischer Verstopfung, mit 17 Jahren wurde eine Magenerkrankung festgestellt. Im Jahr 1892 wurde diese durch eine Behandlung im Präfekturspital kuriert, zwei Jahre später jedoch begann der Magen zu schwellen. »Der Bauchumfang an der breitesten Stelle betrug beim Spitalbesuch 98 cm. Wenn der Patient auf dem Rücken lag, konnte man ganz deutlich eine windende Bewegung im Bauchbereich feststellen. Diese verstärkte sich durch die Berührung mit der Hand, mit etwas Kaltem oder aber auch durch elektrischen Strom. Mit dem Stethoskop hörte man ein tiefes Pochen, und der Bauch fühlte sich an wie ein riesiges Luftkissen«, schreibt der Arzt weiter. »Ungewöhnlich ist, daß Herr Uemori, trotz dieser Symptome eine mehr oder weniger gesunde Verdauung mit einem Stuhlgang pro Tag aufweist.« Als man jedoch den Magen genauer untersuchte, stellte man fest, daß die Menge des Pepsins (Ferment des Magensaftes, das Eiweiß spaltet) normal war. Dr. Kodama vermutete den Grund der Erkrankung in einer mechanischen Dysfunktion im Pylorus, der Verbindung zwischen Magen und Zwölffingerdarm. (S. 85)

1897 berichtet ein Arzt namens Tachisaburo Sarai in »Geibi Iji« von einem Tetanus-Fall mit schwerwiegenden Folgen: Der 24-jährige Mann erkrankte mit neun Jahren an Tetanus (Wundstarrkrampf) und konnte seitdem seinen Unterkiefer nicht mehr bewegen. Die Nahrung nahm er durch die Öffnung, die sich durch das Fehlen von Zähnen ergab, in Breiform ein. Voller Mitleid meinte Dr. Sarai: »Noch nie hat er ein *Manju* (japanisches Brotteig-Plätzchen) gegessen, von Mandarinen kennt er nur den Saft, und Nudeln ißt er, indem er sie mit den Lippen und der Zunge gewissermaßen zerkaut.« Der Patient hatte zwar Mühe zu sprechen, man verstand jedoch ungefähr, was er meinte. Am 24. Dezember 1896 wurde der Gelenkkopf des Unterkiefers auf der rechten Seite durchgetrennt. Die Operation verlief glimpflich: Der Patient mußte wegen einer Zyanose wiederbelebt werden. Zwei Tage später jedoch war seine Aussprache deutlich verbessert, und am 30. Dezember nahm er schon drei Schalen Reis zu sich. Am 20. Januar des folgenden Jahres ging man zur Operation der linken Seite über, die jedoch von weiteren Komplikationen begleitet war. Am 7. April notierte der Arzt, daß sich die rechte Gesichtshälfte mehr oder weniger normalisiert habe. (S. 153)

Dies sind nur drei der Krankengeschichten – von den anderen Patienten kennen wir nur die Gesichter und die Aura, die sie umgibt. Doch jeder einzelne von ihnen hat eine Geschichte zu erzählen: von einem Leben, das sich durch die Krankheit zeitweise oder bleibend verändert hat. Nun liegen sie zusammen mit anderen Menschen als Geheimnisse in dieser Schachtel, vielleicht für immer.

Anna von Senger

THE BOX THAT MY FRIEND showed me was adorned with elegant Japanese letters and of a rare quality. It was kept in the semi-subterranean office of a dealer. The contents of the box confirmed the idea that a certain sadness was inherent in traditional Japanese aesthetics. When I opened the box, I discovered little packets wrapped in cellophane. I opened one of them. It contained images of men, women, and children with unspeakable faces. The box exuded a strange smell, intoxicating but different from alcohol. I was electrified, and before I opened the next packet, I smelled again a photograph that had caught my attention. The photographs conjured up an unreal world—fantastic characters just like in Kabuki theater, and names of diseases you hardly ever hear anymore these days. The people in the photographs were sad, like in Kabuki as I just said, or in the legends that I used to read in illustrated books when I was a child.

This immense document of suffering not only reports the symptoms of diseases, it also represents the everyday life of the patients. Some of them strike rather theatrical poses. The man with the large abscess—maybe he is an artist—makes you wonder whether he was a *kadozuke* (a migrant artist living on alms who performed various tricks and read the sutras in front of the town gates) or a *zato* (the collective name in pre-modern Japan for blind people wearing a monk's attire who played Japanese instruments, like biwa or koto, or gave massages and acupuncture). A woman whose black satin collar suggests the red-light district and whose hair was adorned with a loose hairpin embellished with flowers (did she wear it just for this unique photo-opportunity?) suffered from a large tumor on her neck.

In pre-modern Japan, there was an aesthetic that had a considerably stronger connection to ghosts and phantoms than today's. There were many customs supposed to bring good luck. During absences of the master of the house, people in Tokonoma would hang up the painting of a ghost. In order to ensure their success, storytellers had representations of evil ghosts painted on the linings of their haori dresses. In order to ward off bad luck, some had the image of executed villains (or their heads) painted on their clothes. There were fabulous creatures like the *Zashikiwarashi* that brought wealth to the family they settled with. In summer some tried to attain coolness by daring to enter abandoned buildings or show booths, i.e. "touching" the uncanny and evanescent. Some of these customs you will hardly encounter in any other country.

In Japan, this narrow archipelago in a north-south arc, the finely woven kimono, created with patience, perseverance, skill, and industry, is fitted out with a lining of sadness—the sadness of the demi-monde, the sumo wrestlers, the city dwellers, the daughters of urban families, the factory workers, the showmen, the merchants, the artisans and of many more. Naturally, sadness can be found on the hidden reverse of other countries, too. But it seems to me that particularly in Japan—because of the different moral codes, the countless traditions, and the tried patience of its natives—there is a tendency to rejoice in sadness, maybe in order to still show an appropriate respect for the transient. Here, they love plates with the lonely and sad image of a heron lost amidst snow-covered mountains.

As I have a predilection for the symbolic, I sometimes wish that I had been born in an earlier time. I am also convinced that there is a sadness intrinsic to Japanese aesthetics that is not sufficiently described by *wabi* and *sabi,* the terms usually used in this context.

The disappearance of many diseases is certainly a pleasant development. On the other hand, the strange beauty evoked by these images moved me tremendously. I hope that the reader will be moved by a sadness as intense as the one I felt when I first looked at them. And I hope that he or she will surmise the hidden reverse of the Japanese aesthetics once embedded in daily life.

Akimitsu Naruyama

DIE SCHACHTEL, DIE MIR EIN BEKANNTER zeigte, war mit solch stilvollen japanischen Schriftzeichen verziert und von einer solchen Beschaffenheit, wie ich sie kaum je gesehen hatte. Sie wurde im halbunterirdischen Büro eines Händlers aufbewahrt. Der Inhalt der Schachtel bestätigte die Vorstellung, daß der traditionellen japanischen Ästhetik Traurigkeit innewohnt. Beim Öffnen der Schachtel kamen in Zellophanpapier eingewickelte Bündel zum Vorschein, und als ich eines auspackte, erblickte ich Bilder von Männern, Frauen und Kindern mit unsagbaren Antlitzen. Die Schachtel verströmte einen seltsamen Geruch, der – freilich anders als Alkohol – betrunken machte. Ich war aufgeregt, und bevor ich das nächste Bündel öffnete, roch ich noch einmal an einer Fotografie, die mir ins Auge gesprungen war. Eine unwirkliche Welt erschien mir – phantastische Figuren wie aus dem Kabuki-Theater, und Namen von Krankheiten, die man heute kaum mehr hört. Auf den Fotografien waren traurige Menschen zu sehen, wie aus dem Kabuki-Theater eben oder aus Sagen, die ich als Kind in Bilderbüchern las.

Diese immense Chronik des Leidens zeigt nicht nur Krankheitssymptome, sondern auch den Alltag der Patienten. Angesichts der theatralischen Posen, die einige einnehmen, könnte man etwa von dem Mann mit der großen Geschwulst, der wie ein Künstler wirkt, vermuten, daß er ein sogenannter *Kadozuke* war (ein bettelnder Wanderkünstler, der vor den Toren der Häuser verschiedene Künste darbot und Sutren vorlas) oder ein *Zato* (Sammelbegriff für Blinde in Mönchsgewand, die im vormodernen Japan japanische Instrumente wie die Biwa oder Koto spielten oder Massagen und Akupunktur anboten). Eine Frau, die mit ihrem schwarzen Satinkragen aus dem Vergnügungsviertel zu stammen scheint und ihr Haupt mit einer blumenverzierten, losen Haarnadel schmückte (angesichts der einmaligen Gelegenheit, fotografiert zu werden?), trägt an ihrem Hals einen großen Tumor.

Im vormodernen Japan herrschte eine Ästhetik, die viel mehr als die heutige dem Umgang mit Geistern und Gespenstern verpflichtet war. Es gab zahlreiche glücksbringende Bräuche: Wenn der Herr außer Haus war, wurde in Tokonoma, um Unglück abzuwenden, eine Bildrolle mit Gespenstern aufgehängt. Um erfolgreich zu sein, ließen sich Geschichtenerzähler auf die Innenseite ihres Haori-Gewandes böse Geister malen. Um Unheil abzuwenden, ließ man sich ein Bild von

Hingerichteten oder deren Kopf auf die Kleider malen. Es gab Sagengestalten wie das *Zashikiwarashi*, das der Familie, bei der es sich niederließ, Wohlstand brachte. Im Sommer wiederum versuchte man, sich durch Mutproben in verlassenen Gebäuden und Schaubuden zu kühlen, durch das »Berühren« von Unheimlichem und Flüchtigem. Einige dieser Bräuche wird man in anderen Ländern kaum finden.

In Japan, diesem sich von Nord nach Süd erstreckendem, schmalen Inselbogen, hat man den feingewobenen, mit Geduld, Ausdauer, Kraft und Fleiß angefertigten Kimono gleichsam mit einem Innenfutter aus Traurigkeit versehen – jener Traurigkeit der Halbwelt, der Sumo-Ringer, der Städter, der Töchter städtischer Familien, der Fabrikarbeiter, der Schausteller, der Händler, der Handwerker und vieler anderer mehr. Natürlich wird auch in anderen Ländern Traurigkeit auf der verborgenen Innenseite zu finden sein. In Japan aber scheint mir – aufgrund der andersartigen Moral, der zahlreichen Traditionen und der geprüften Geduld der Bewohner – ganz besonders die Neigung zu herrschen, sich an Traurigkeit zu erfreuen, vielleicht um nichtsdestotrotz dem Vergänglichen gebührenden Respekt zu erweisen. Hier herrscht eine Vorliebe für Teller mit dem traurigen Motiv eines Reihers, der sich einsam in den Bergen einer Schneelandschaft verliert.

Da ich einen Hang zum Symbolischen habe, wünsche ich mir manchmal, daß ich in einer früheren Zeit geboren worden wäre. Auch bin ich zur Überzeugung gelangt, daß die Traurigkeit, die der traditionellen japanischen Ästhetik innewohnt, mit den in diesem Zusammenhang häufig verwendeten Begriffen *Wabi* und *Sabi* kaum ausreichend bezeichnet wird.

Daß sich heute viele Krankheiten auf dem Rückzug befinden, ist zweifelsohne ein erfreulicher Umstand. Auf der anderen Seite jedoch hat mich die seltsame Schönheit, die aus diesen Bildern spricht, stark berührt. Ich hoffe, daß der Leser beim Betrachten dieser medizinischen Fotografien von einer ähnlich heftigen Traurigkeit ergriffen wird, wie ich sie empfand, als ich sie zum ersten Mal sah, und so die verborgene Kehrseite der einst im alltäglichen Leben eingebetteten japanischen Ästhetik erahnen wird.

Akimitsu Naruyama

PLATES

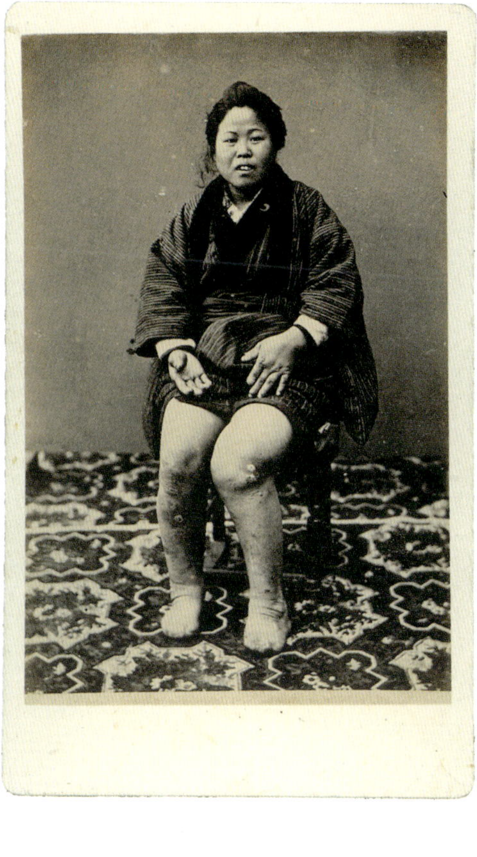

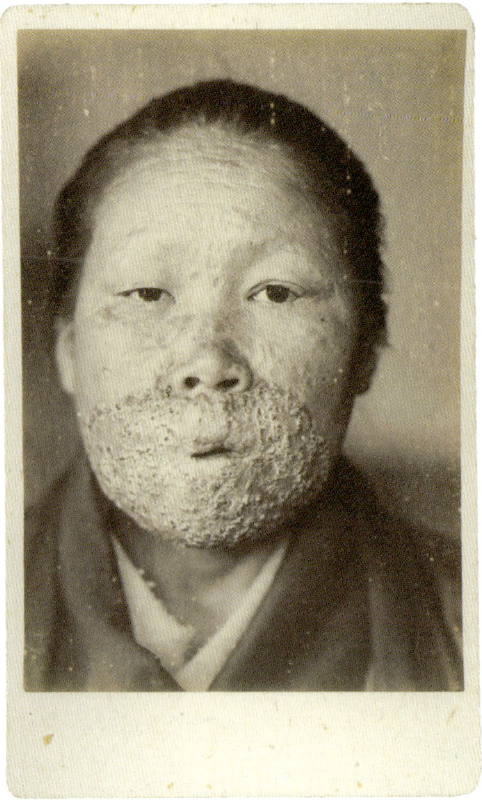

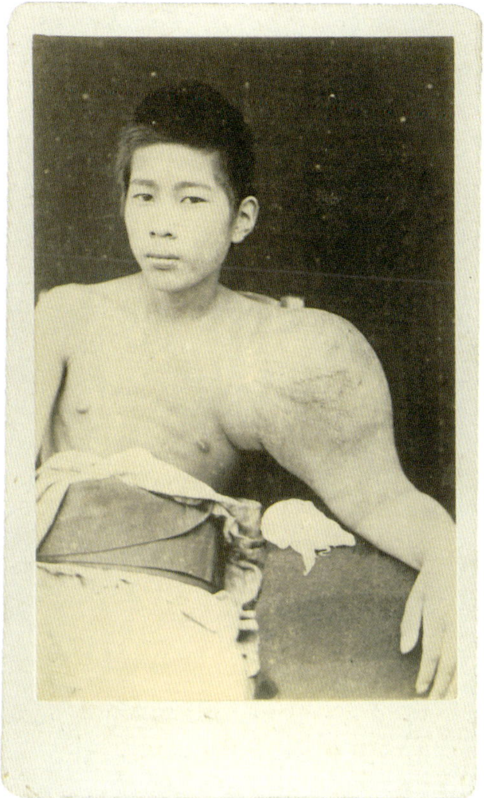

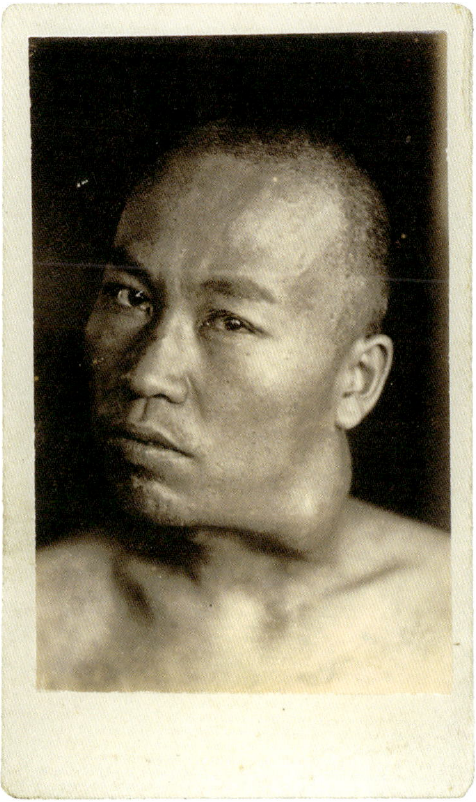

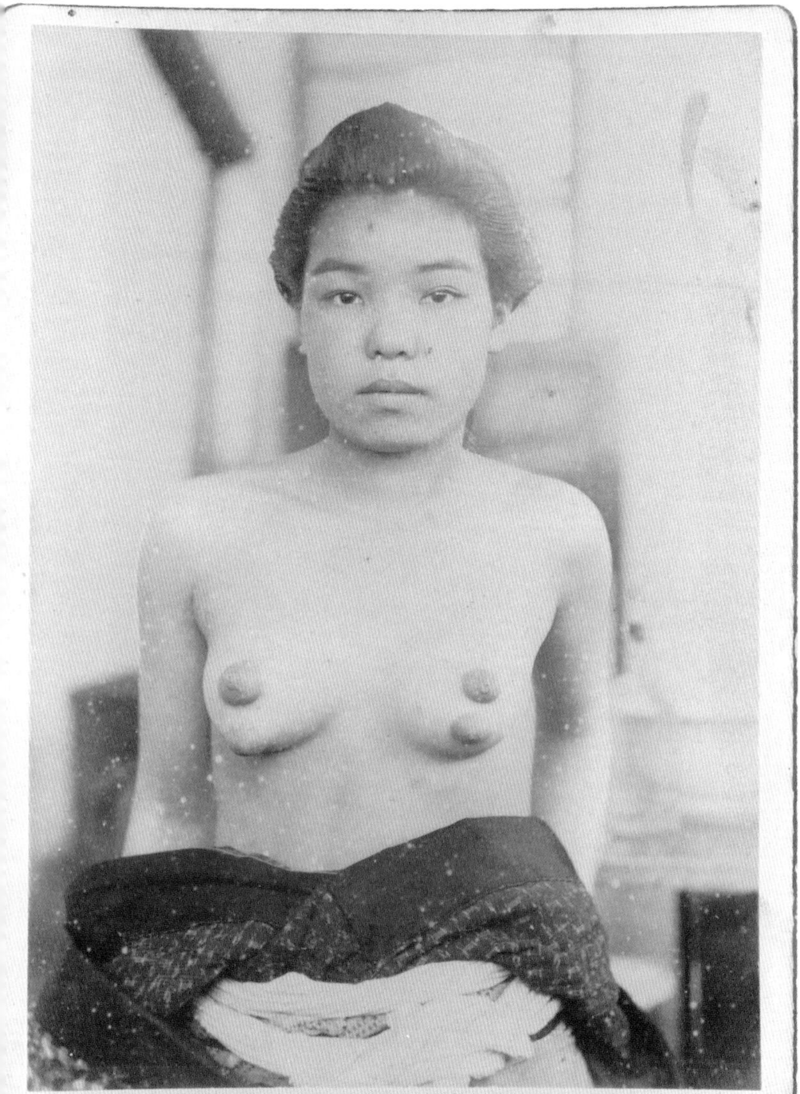

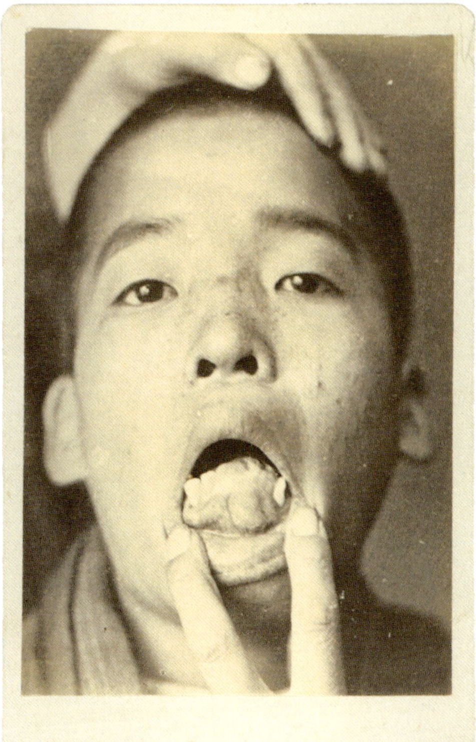

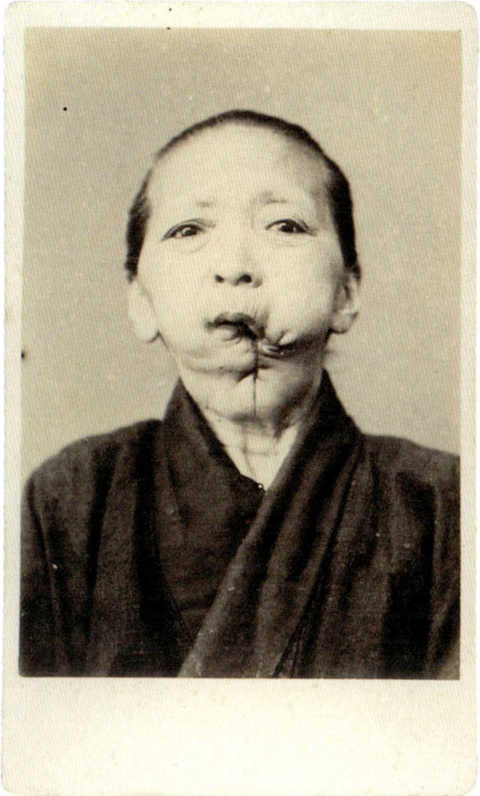

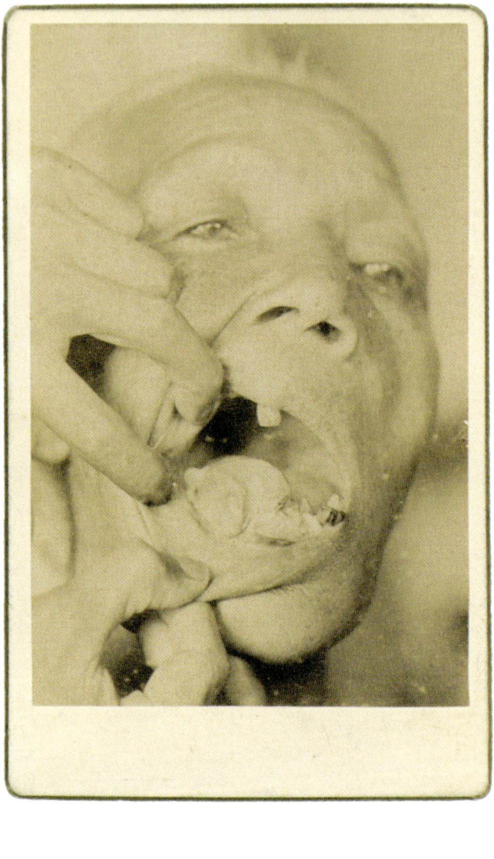

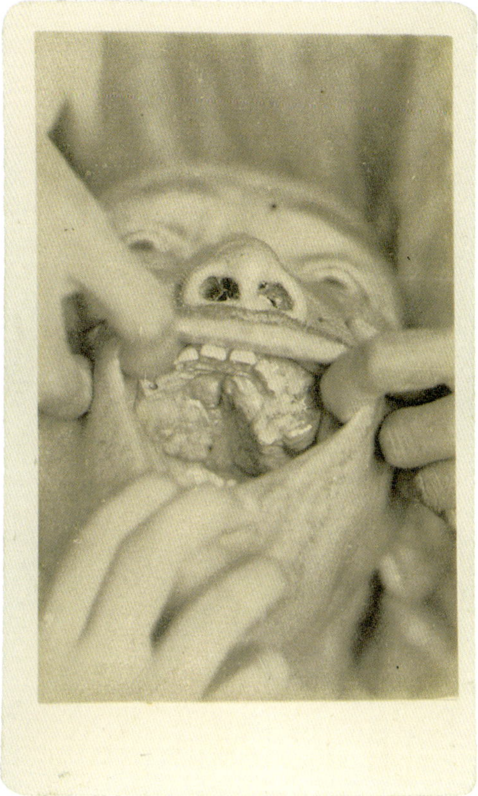

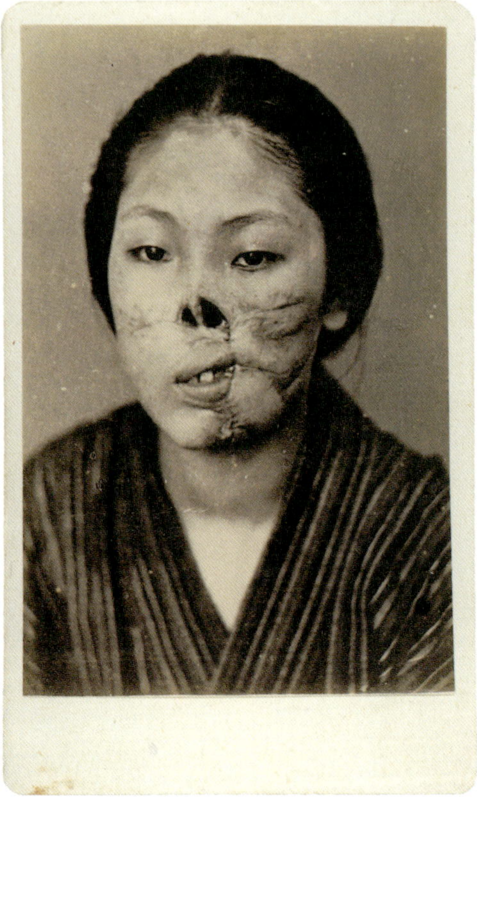

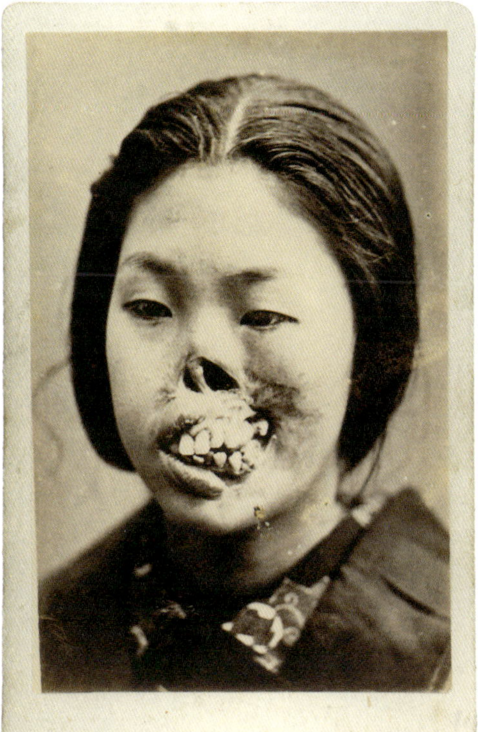

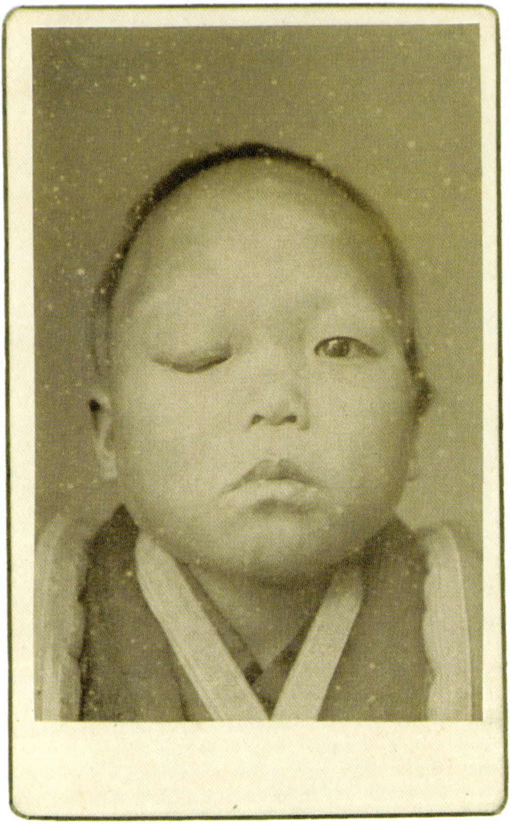

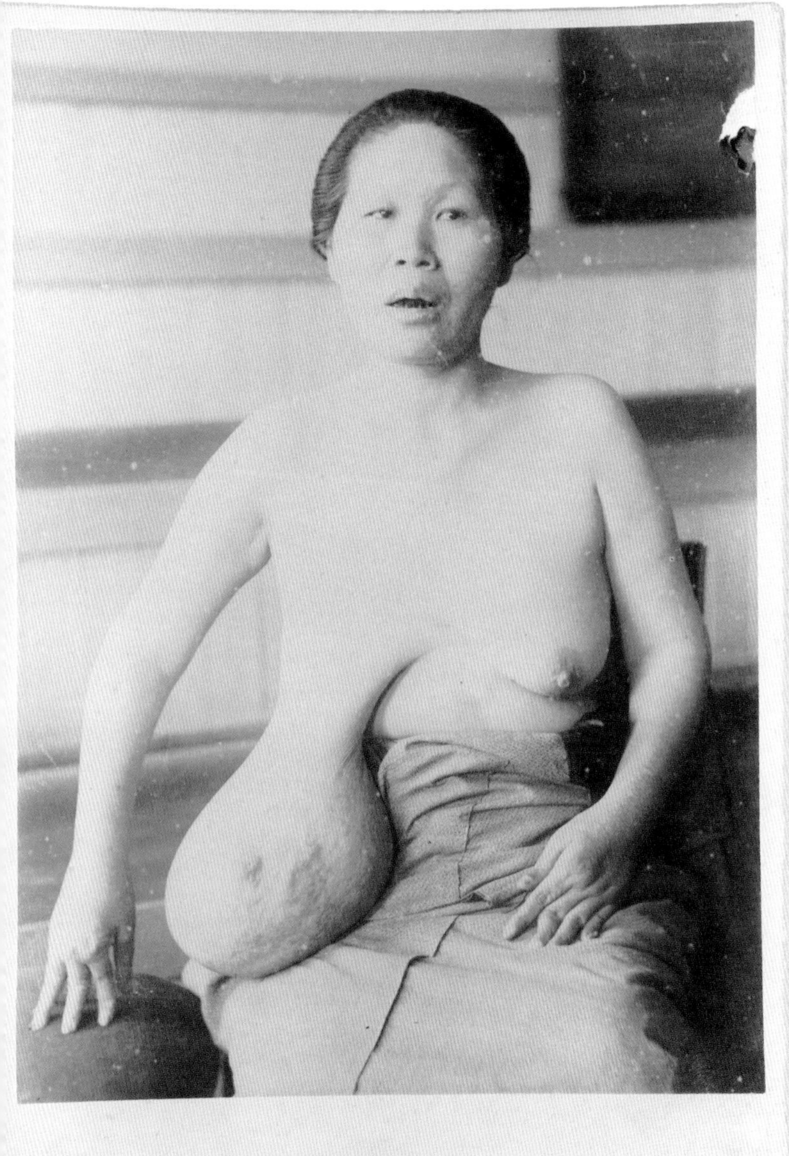

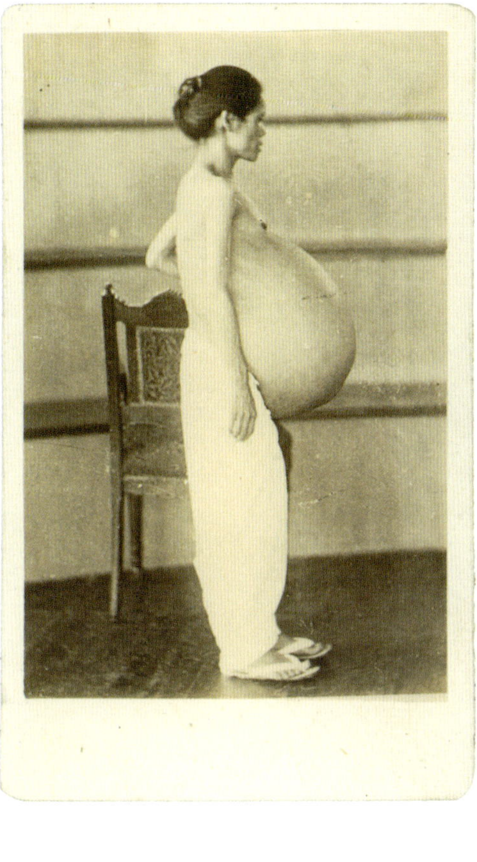

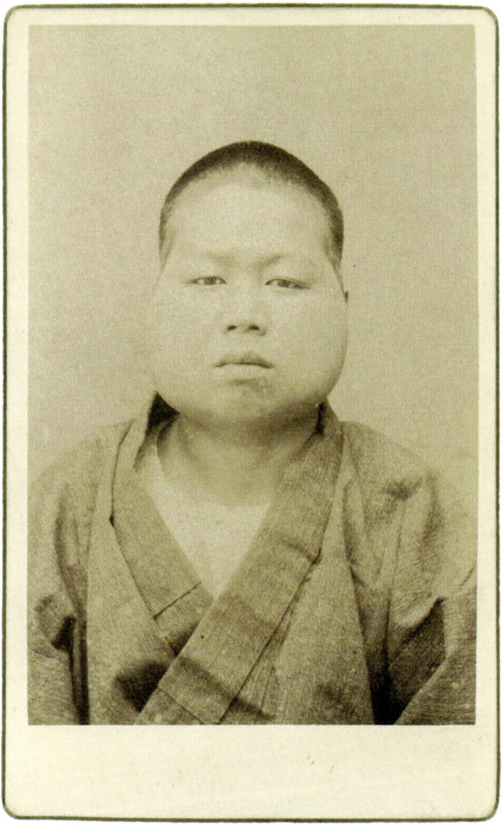

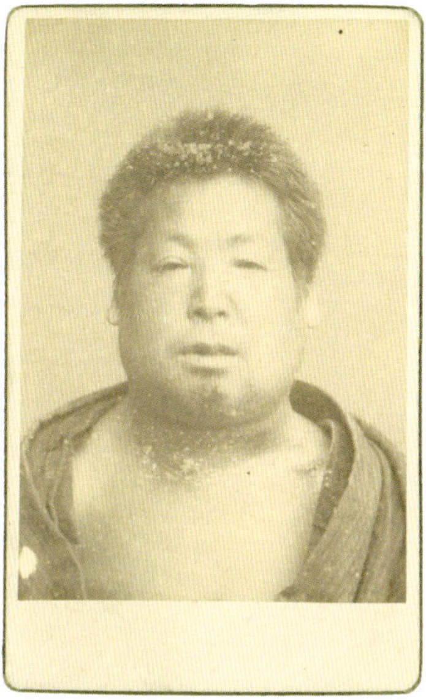

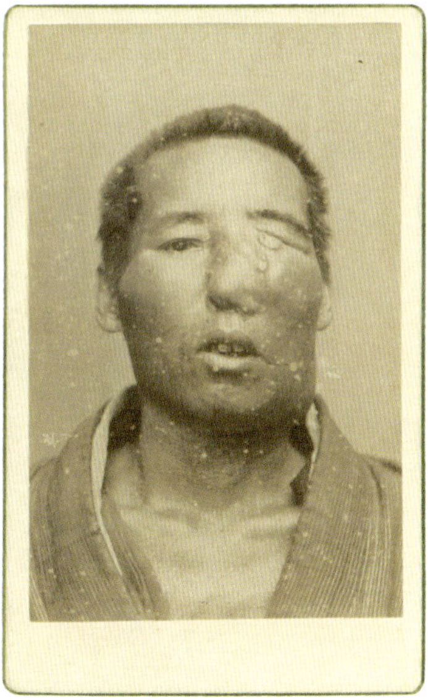

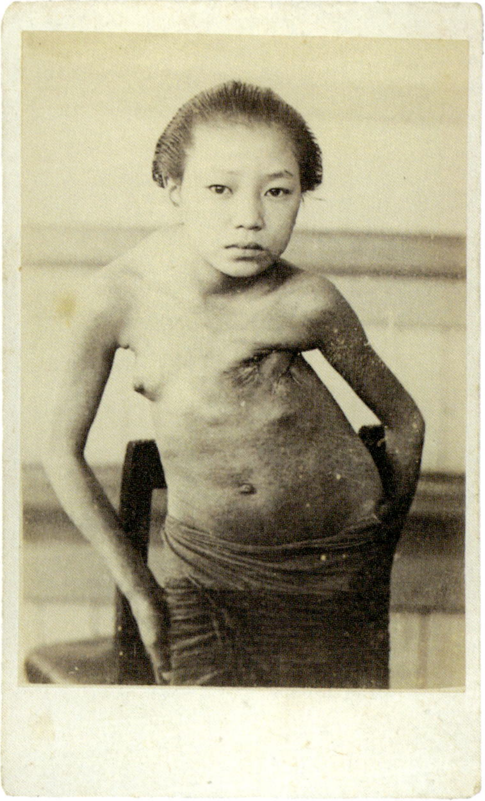

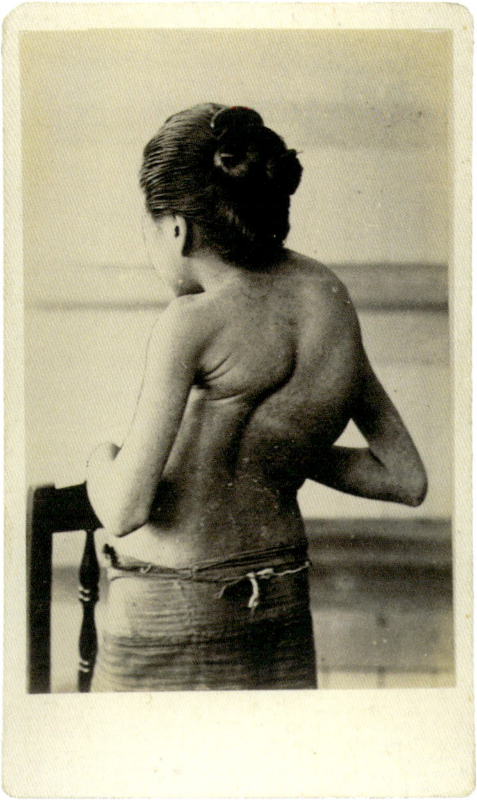

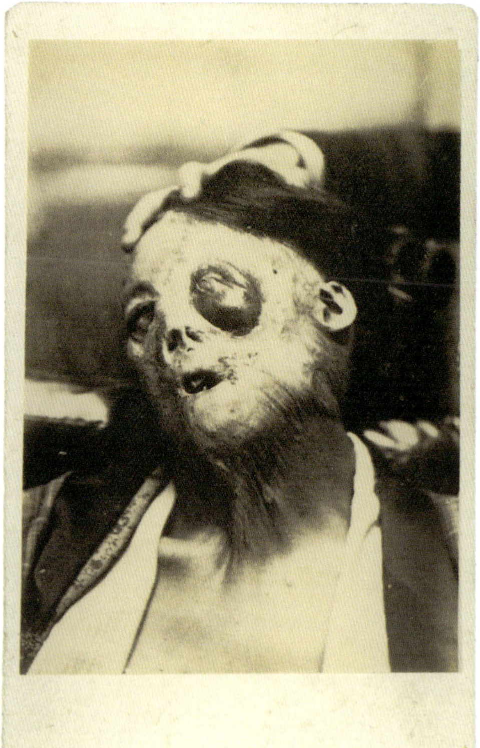

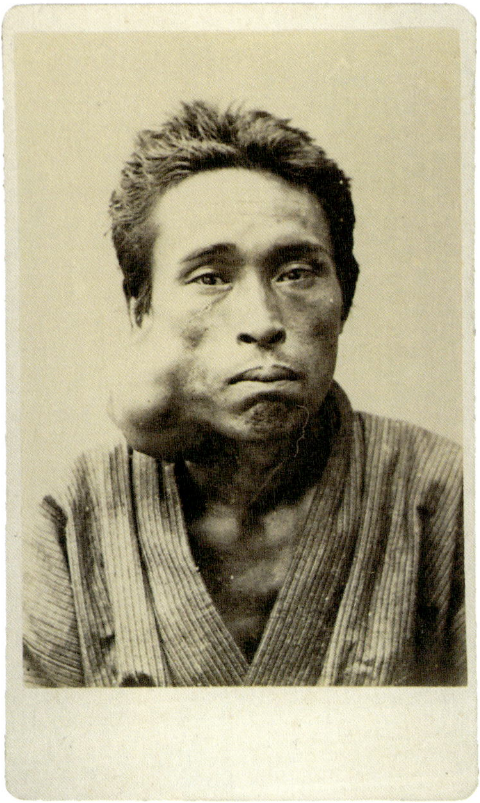

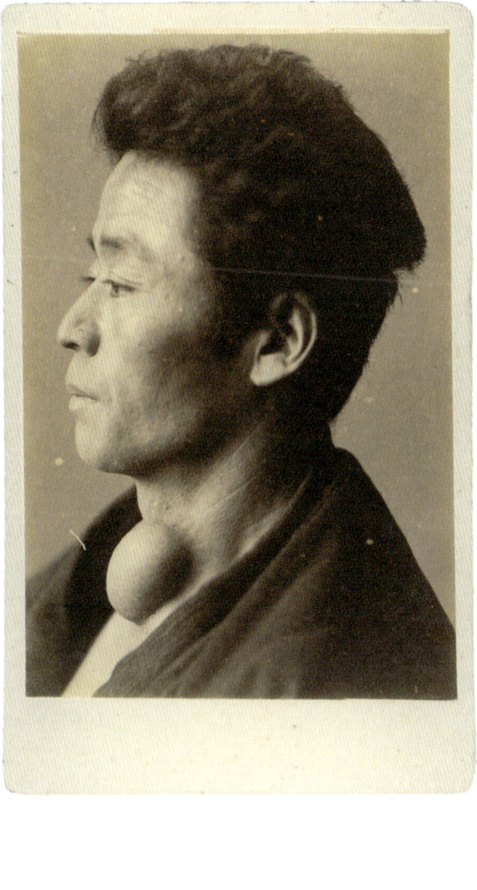

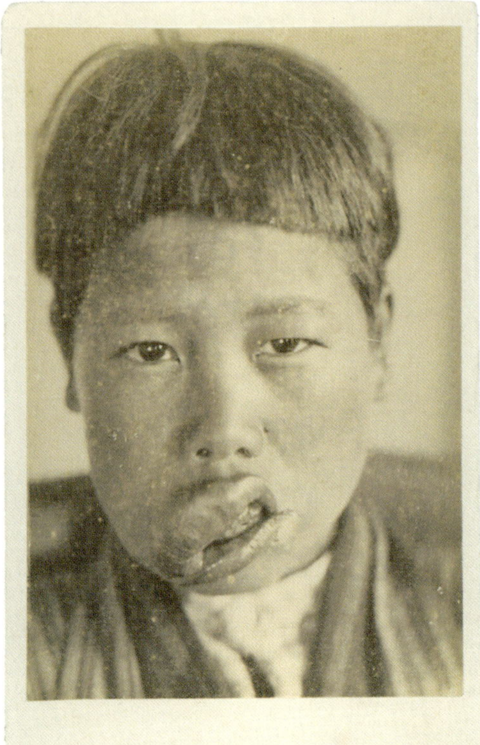

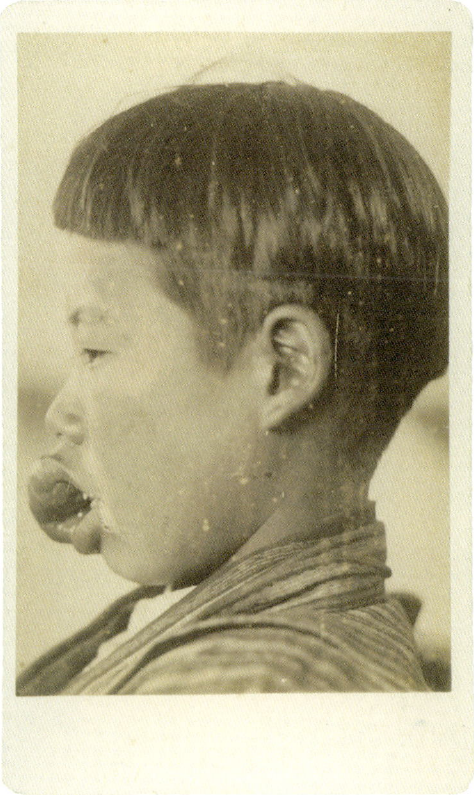

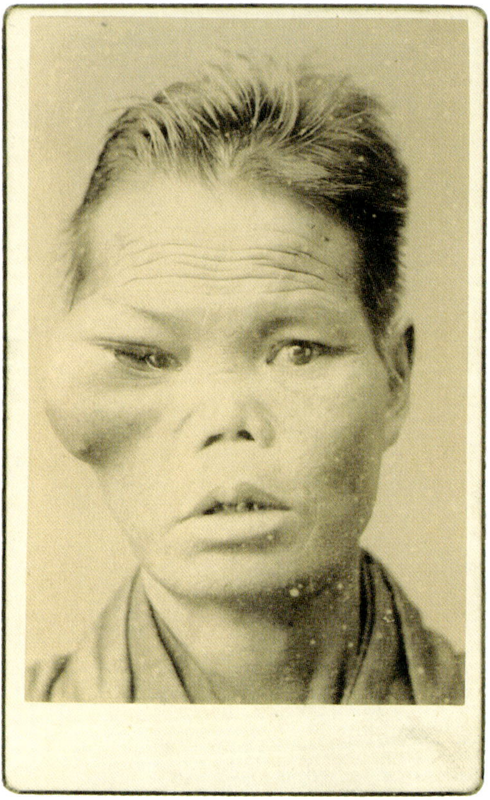

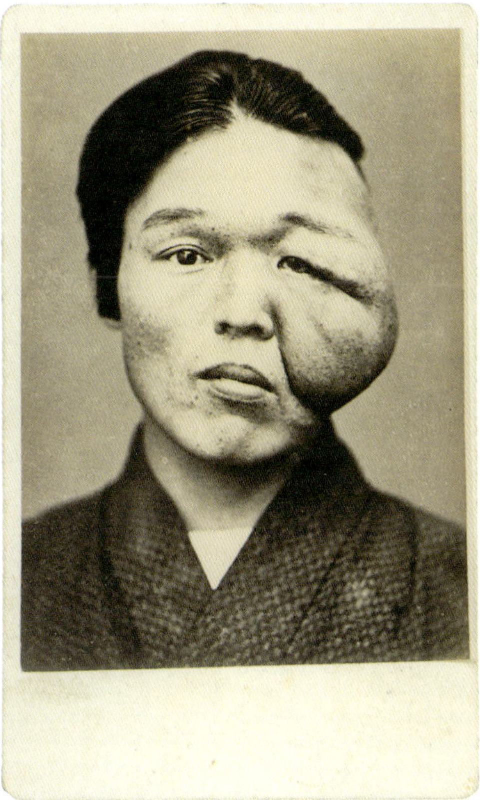

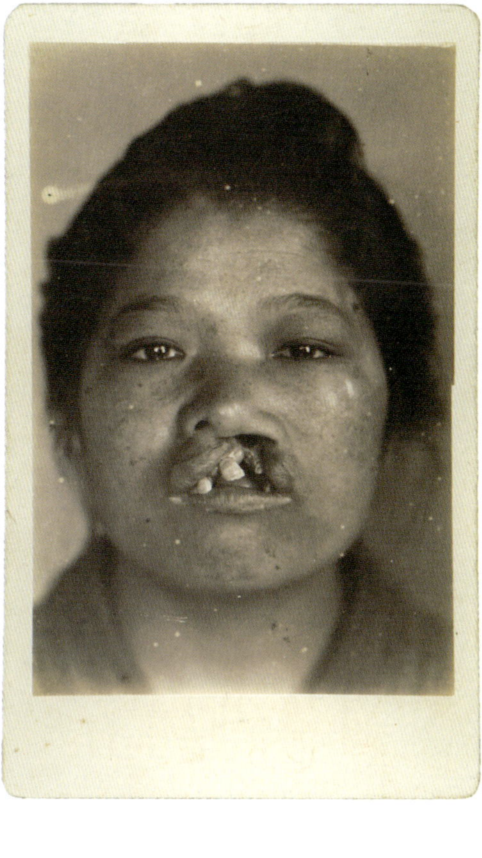

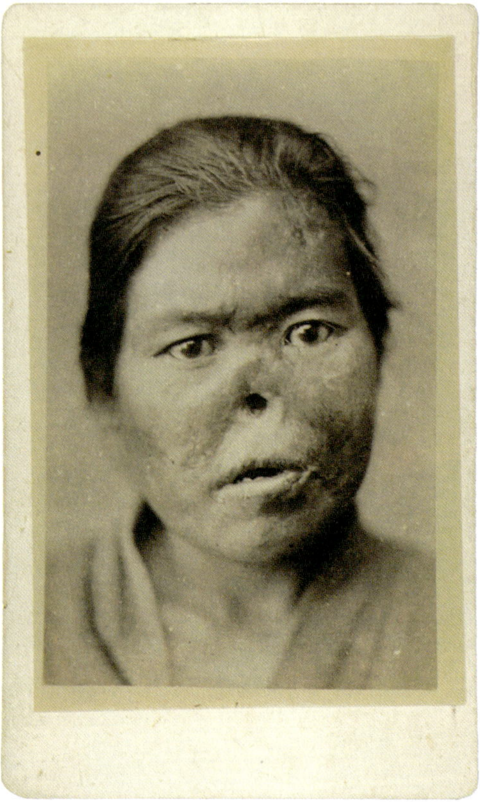

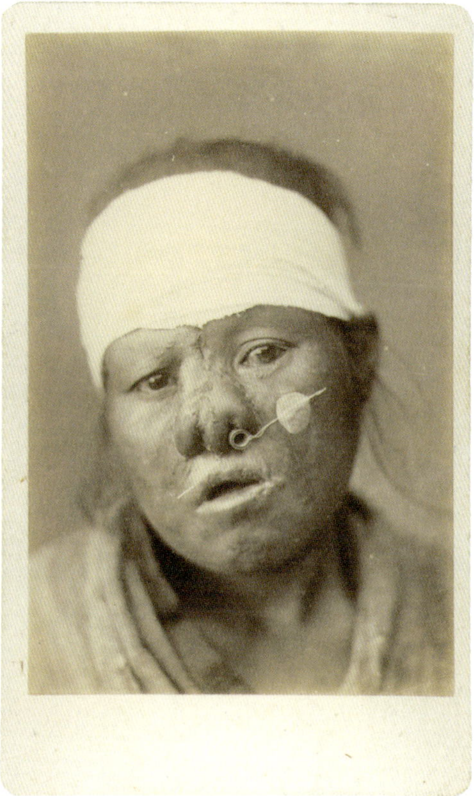

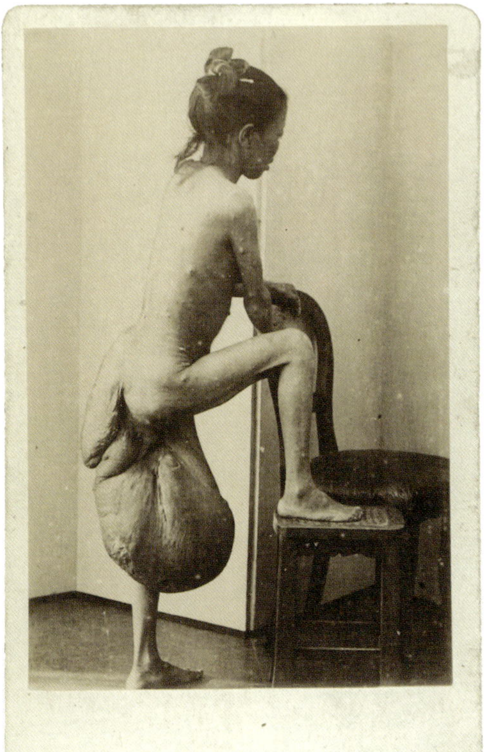

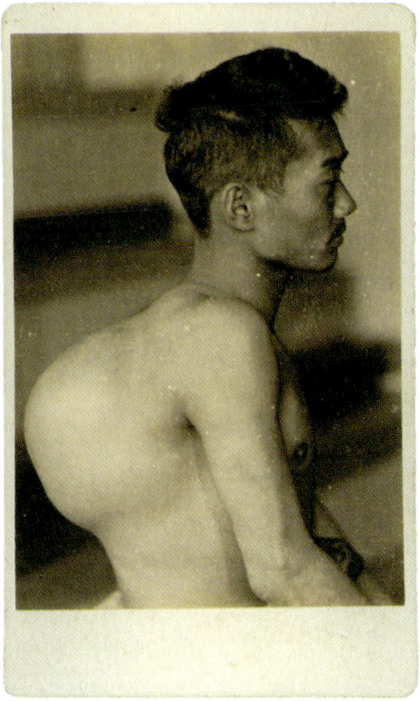

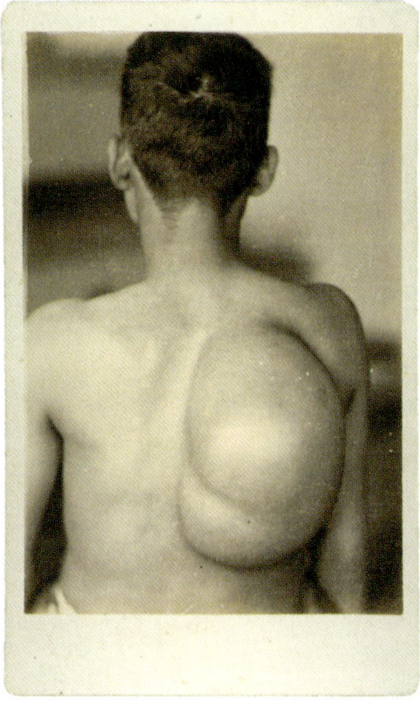

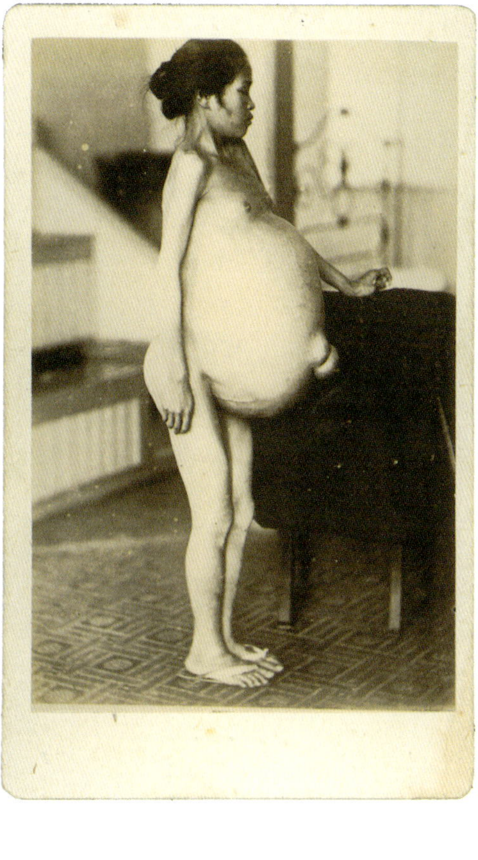

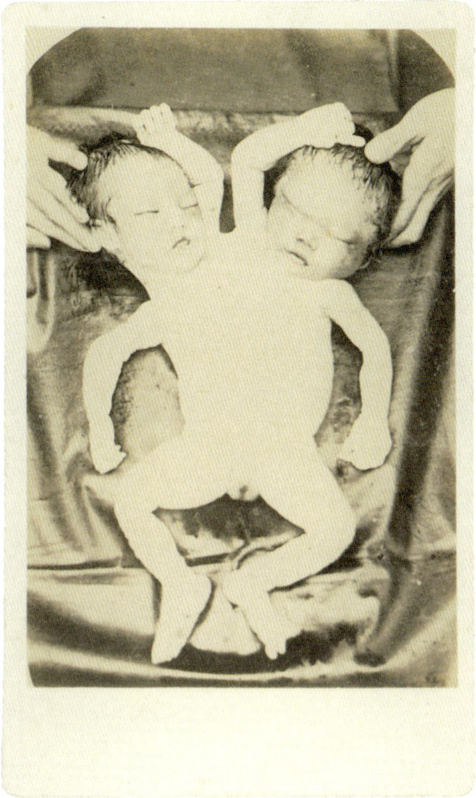

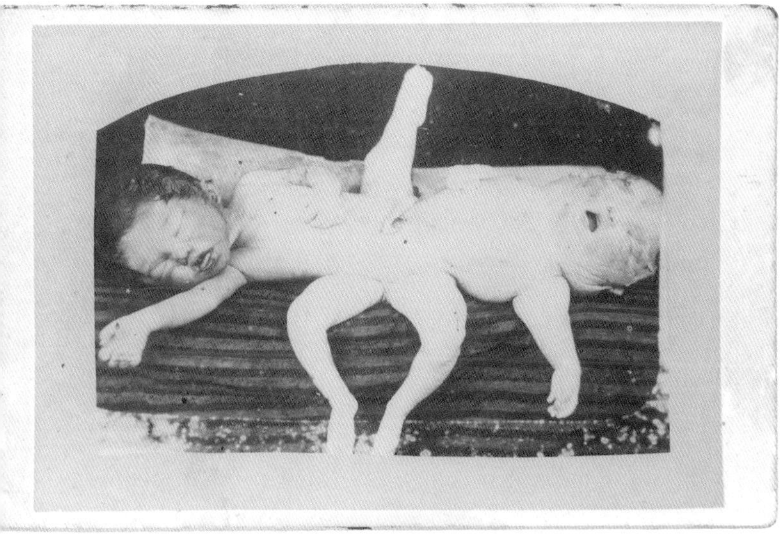

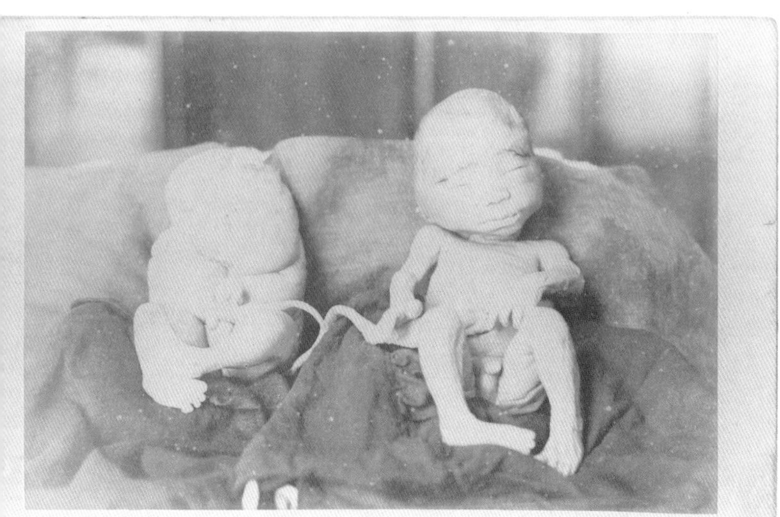

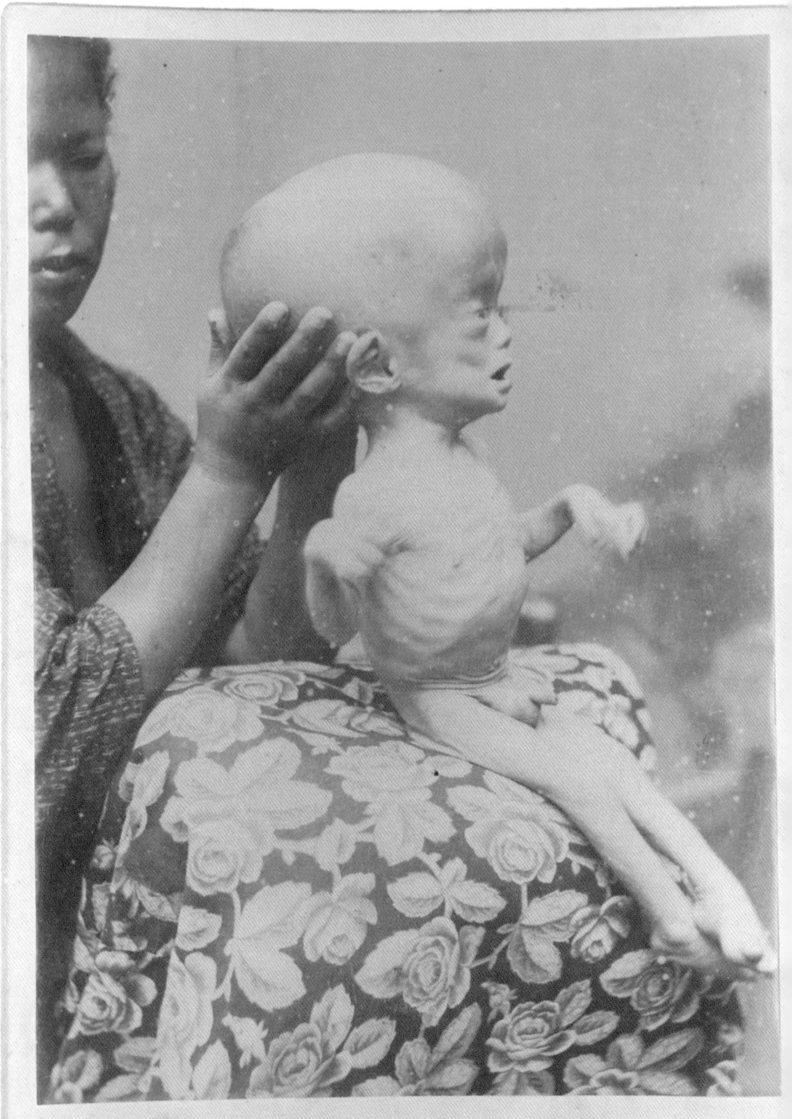

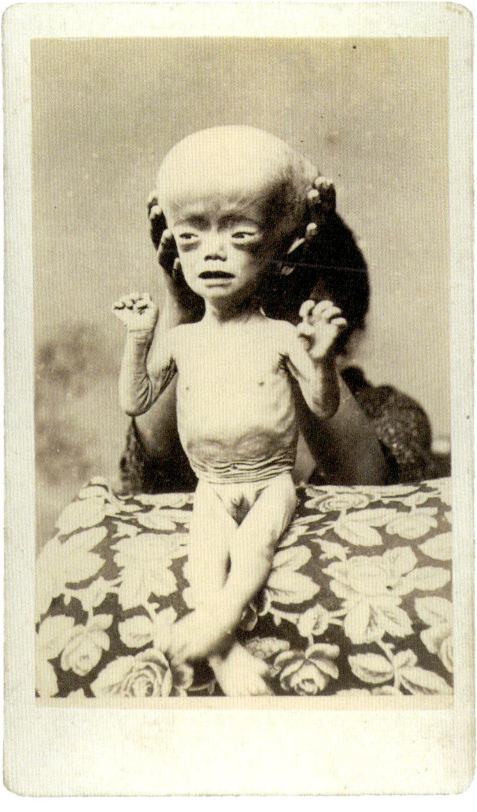

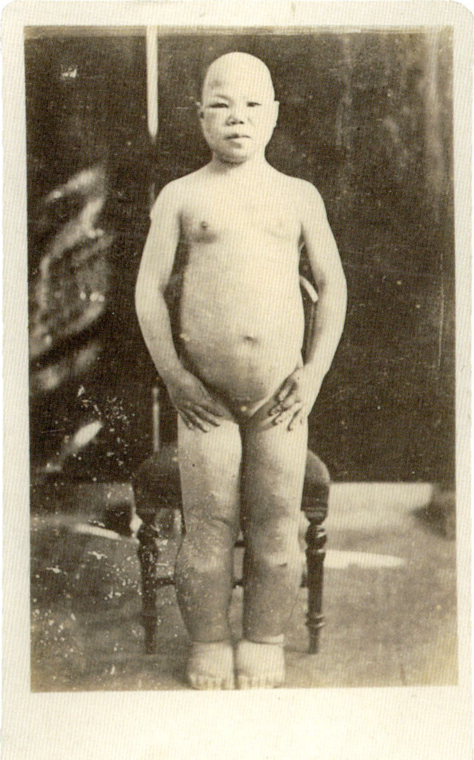

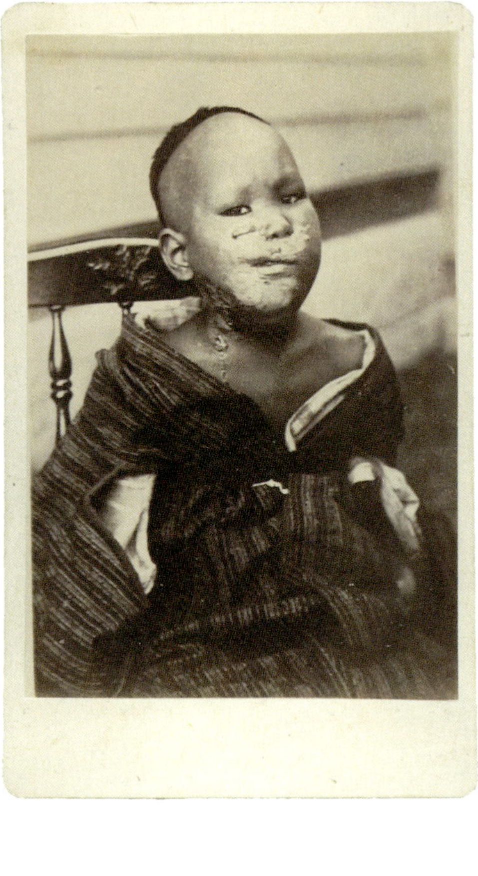

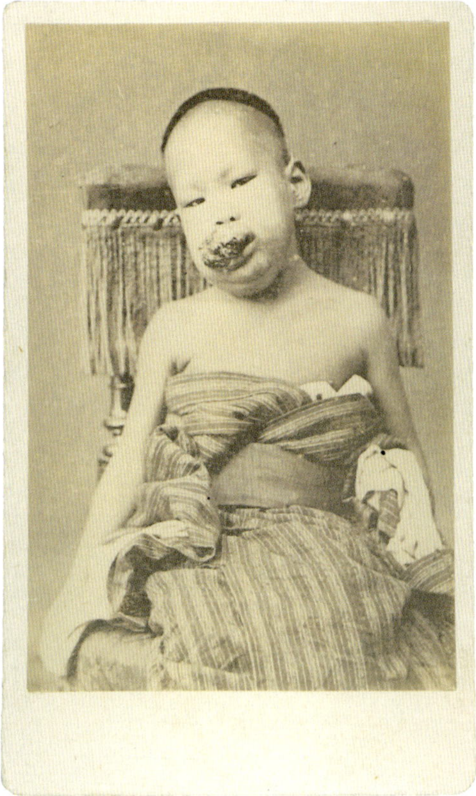

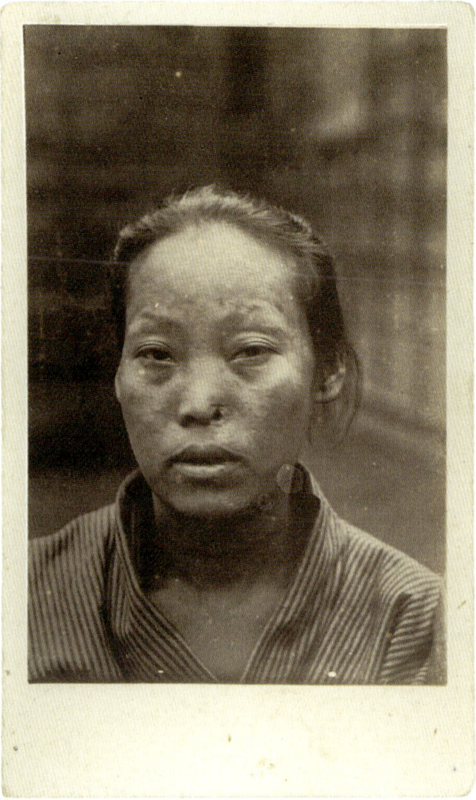

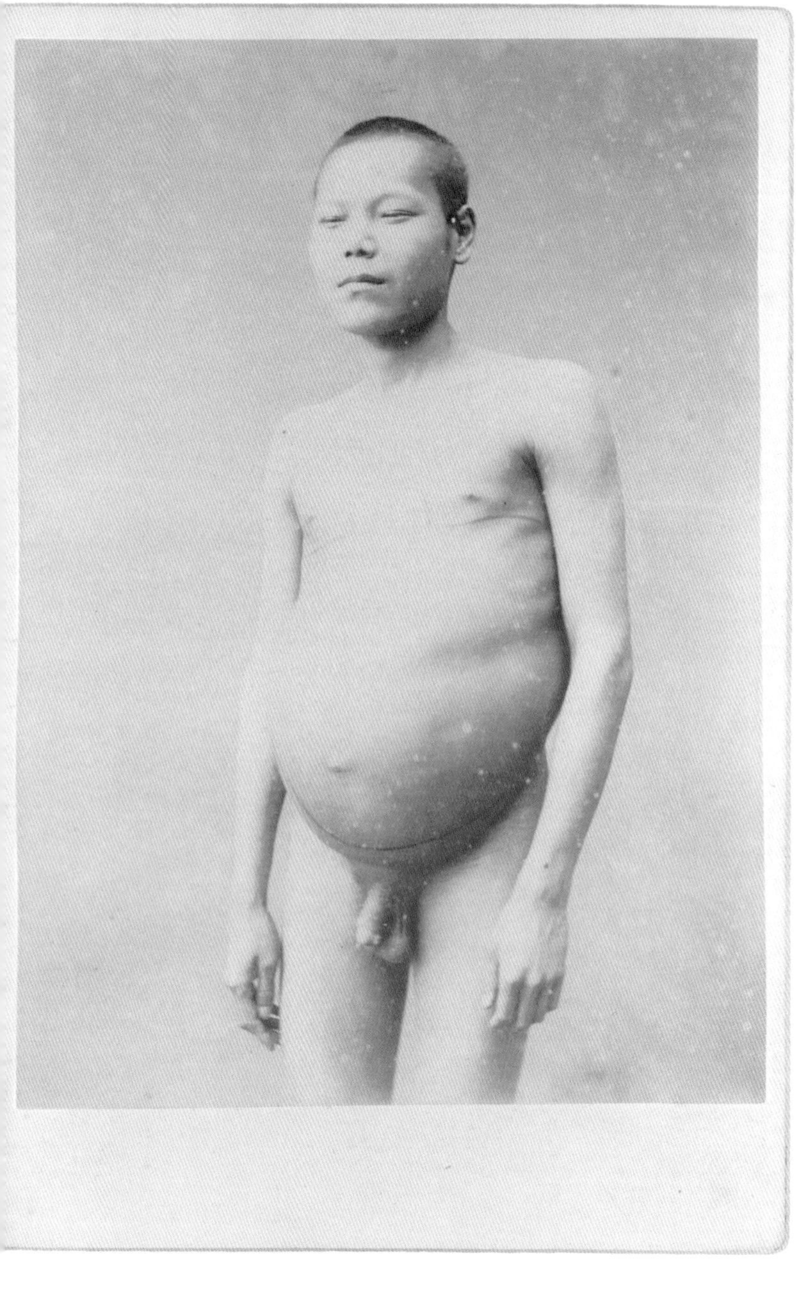

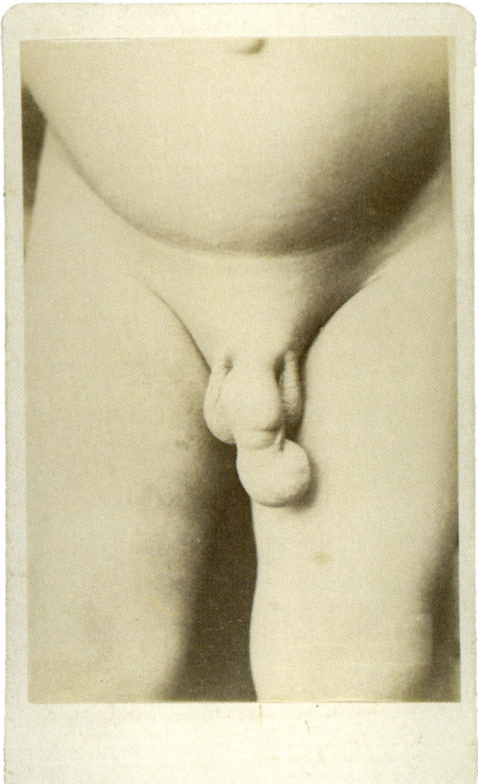

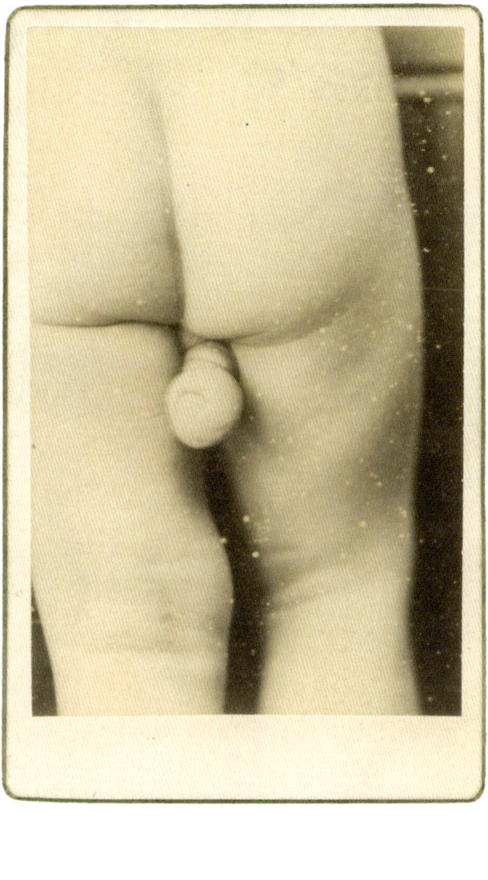

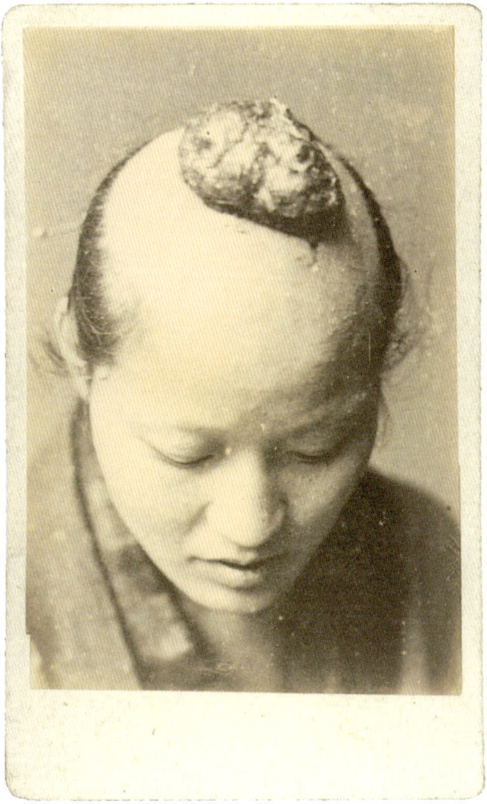

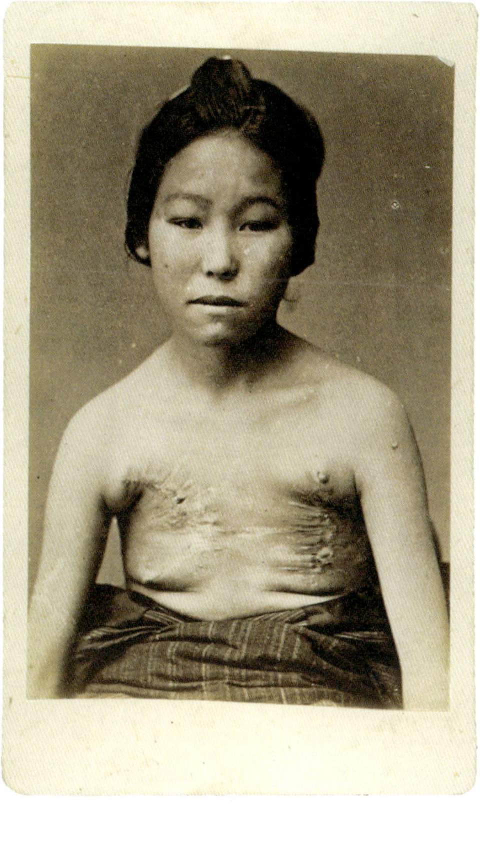

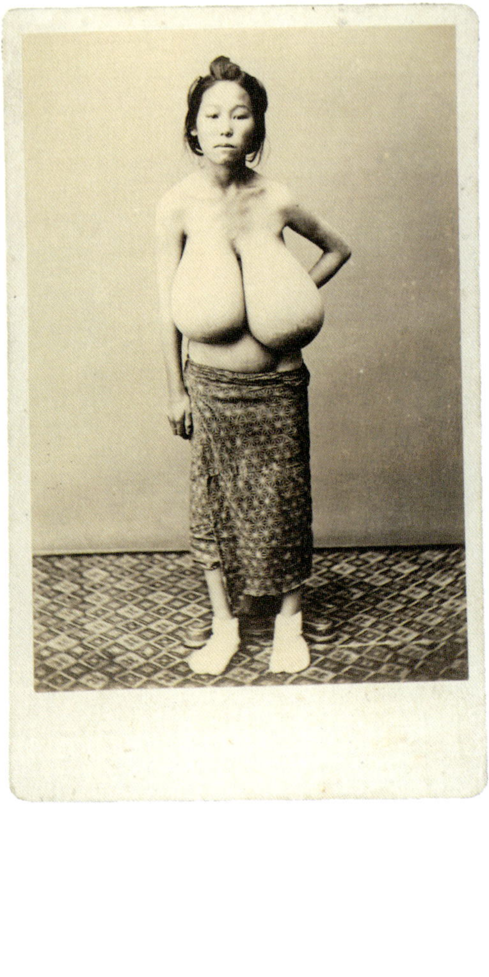

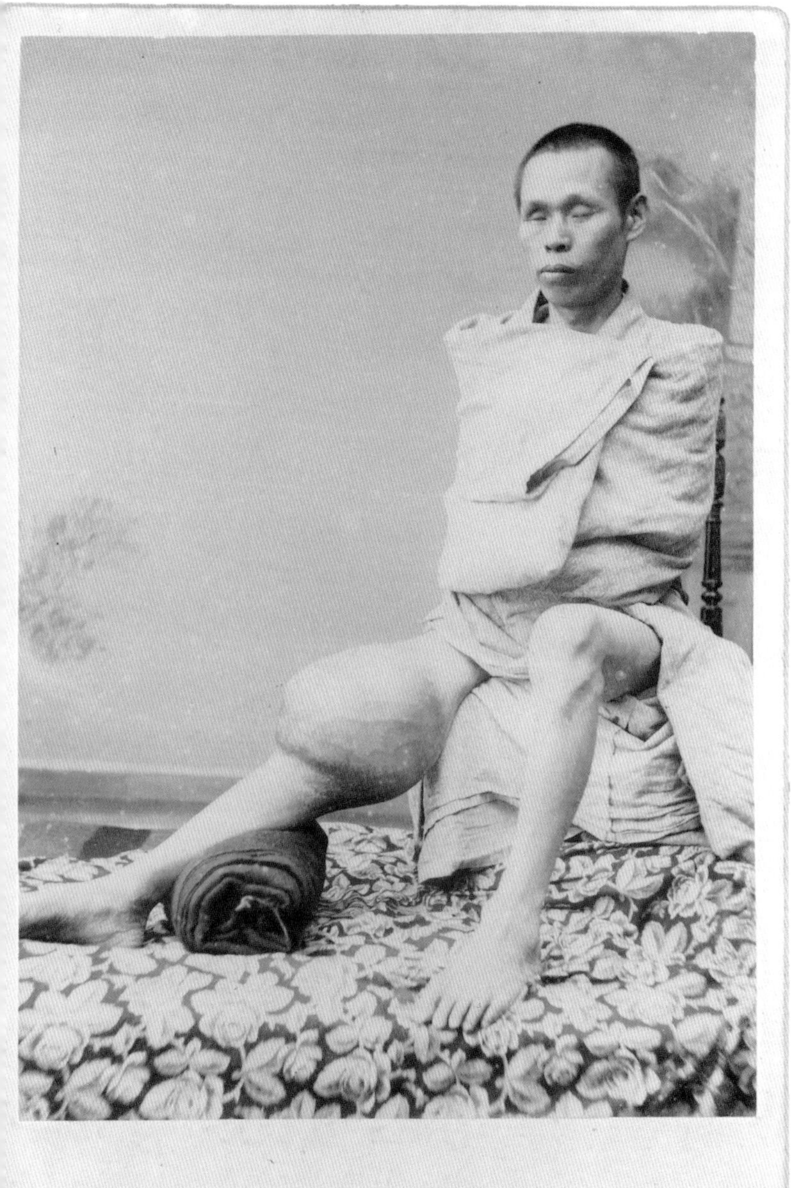

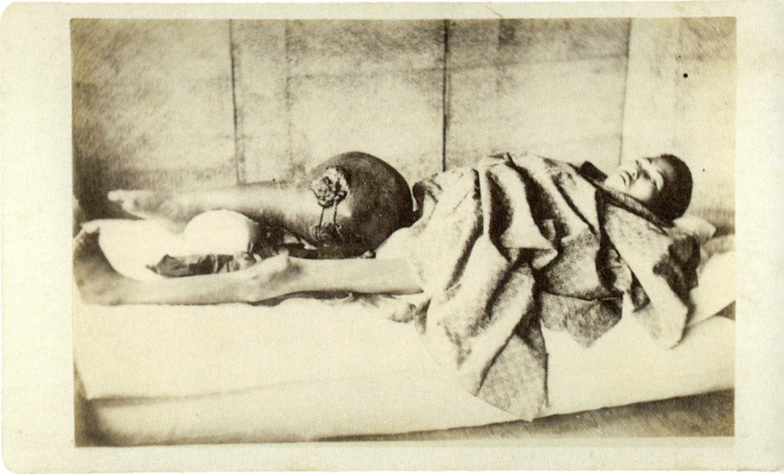

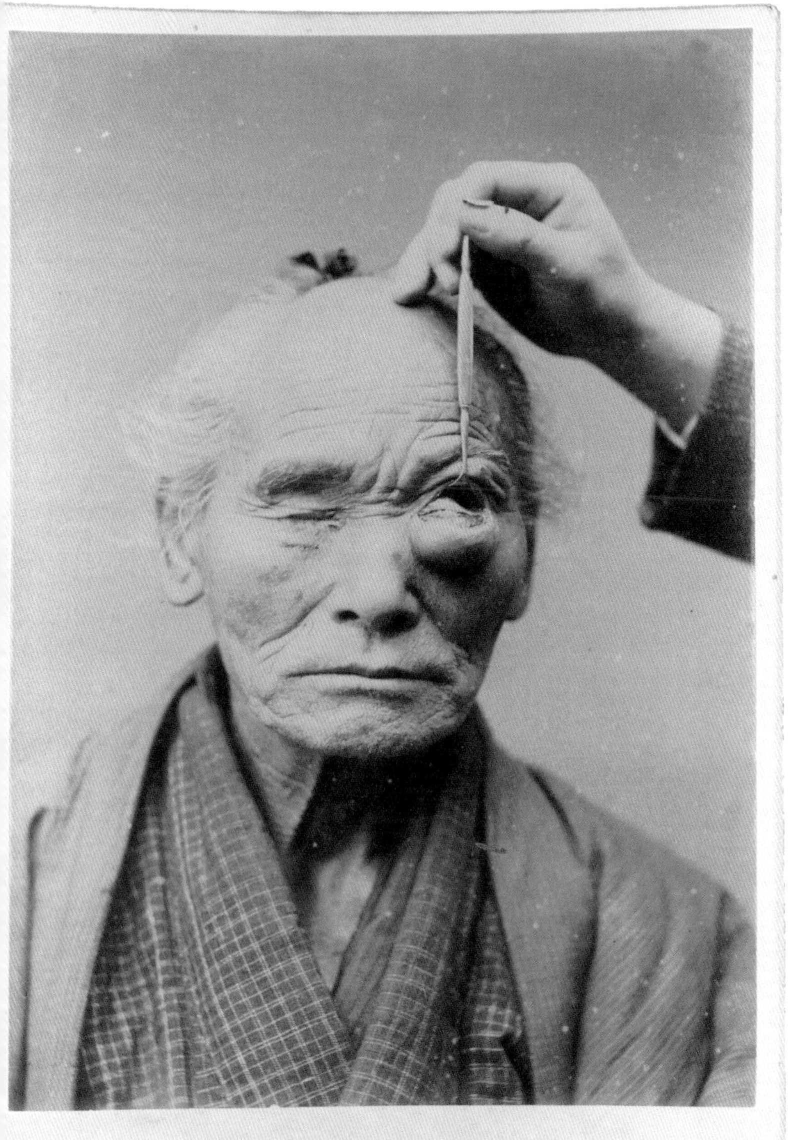

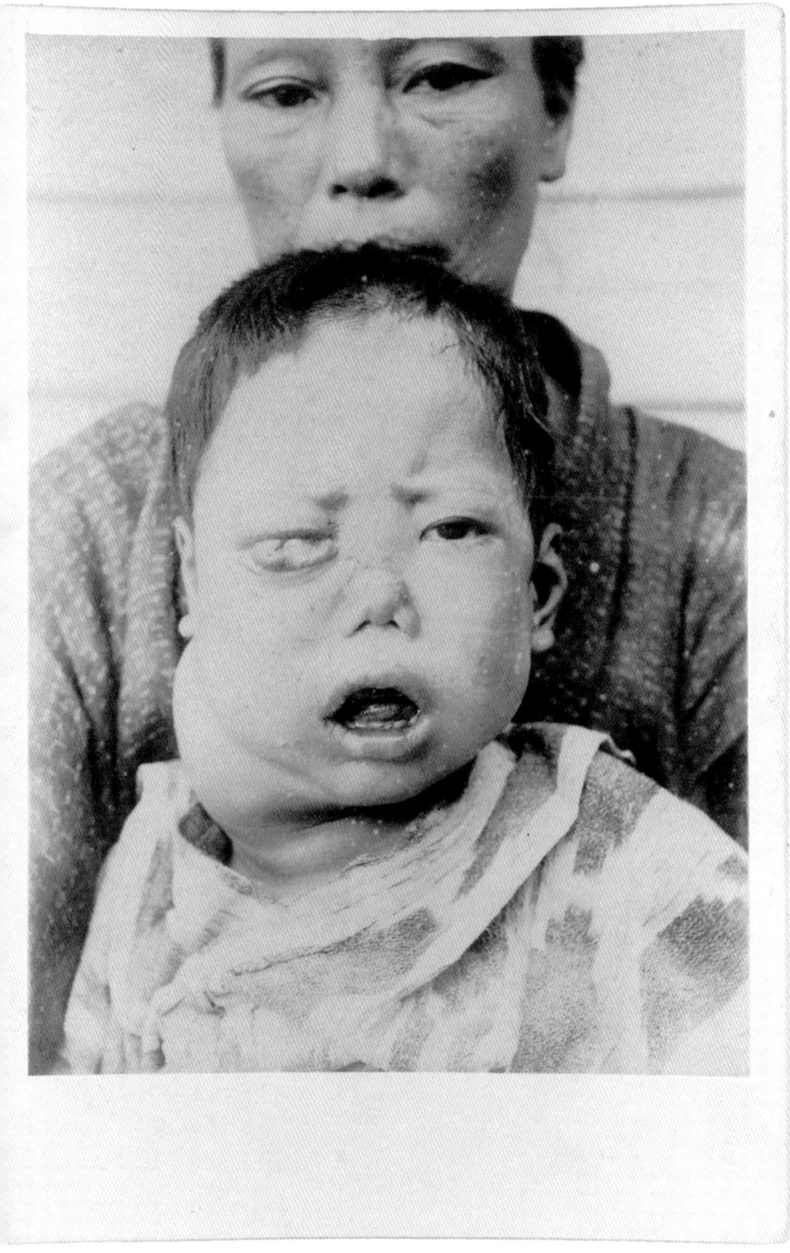

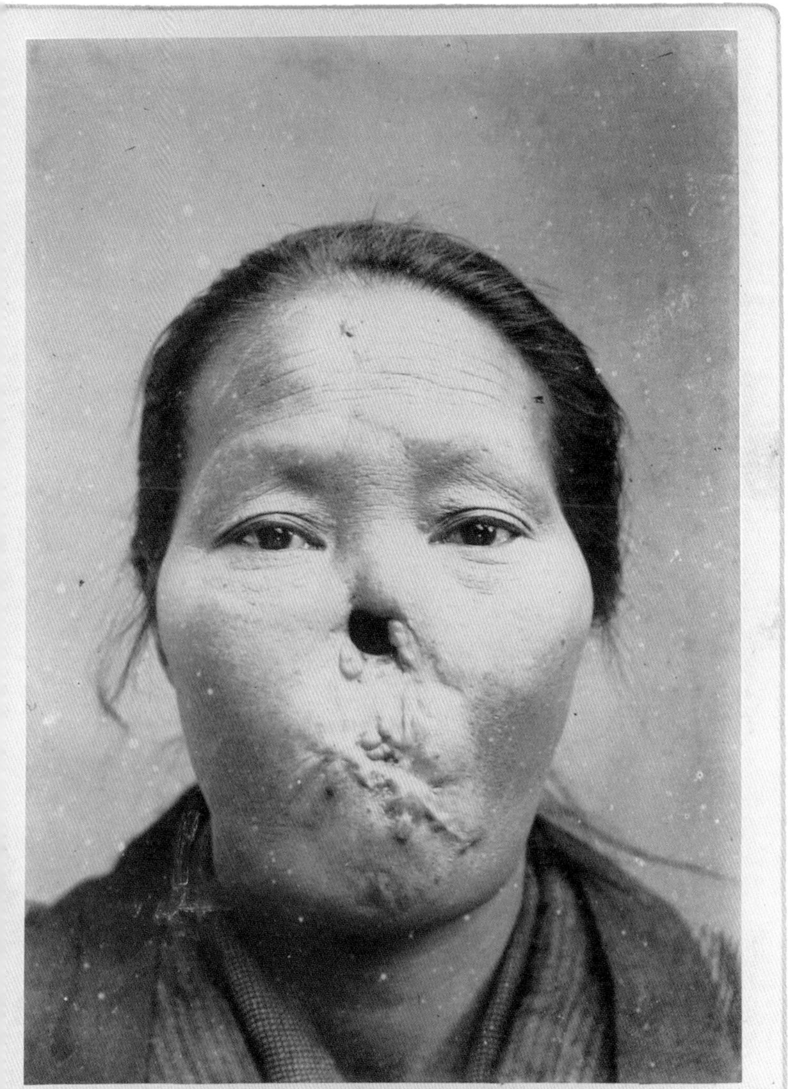

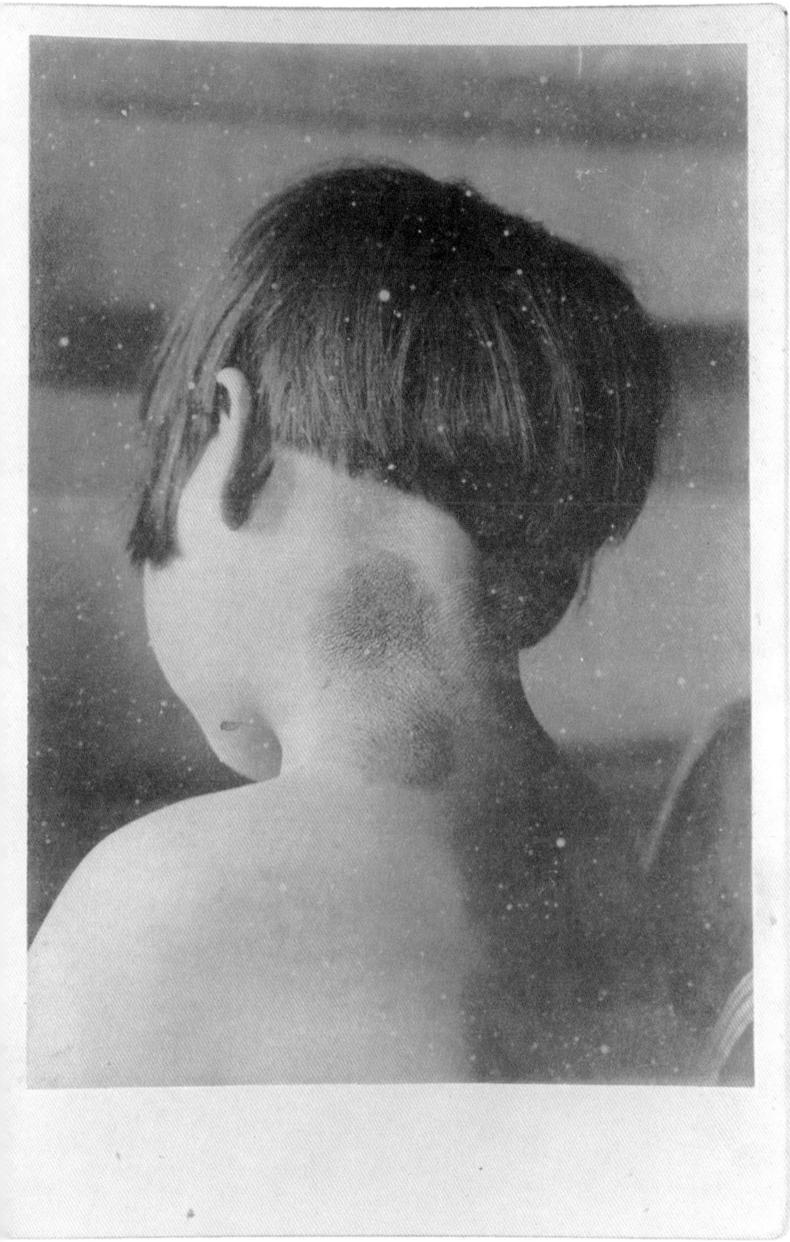

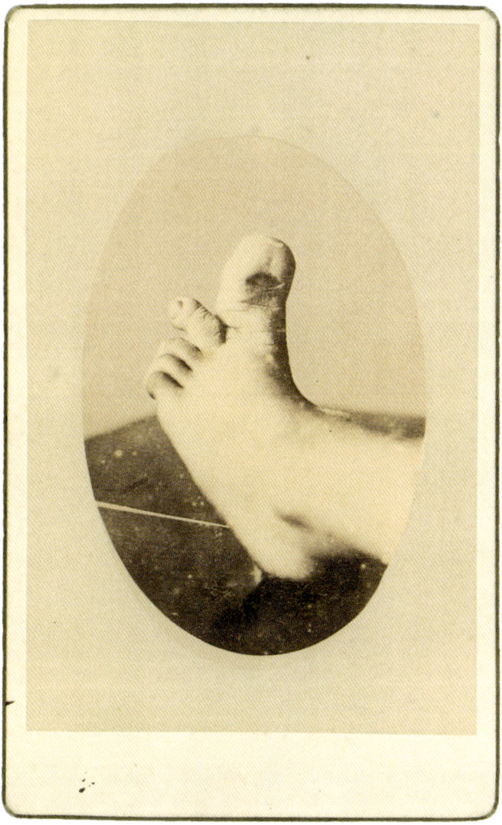

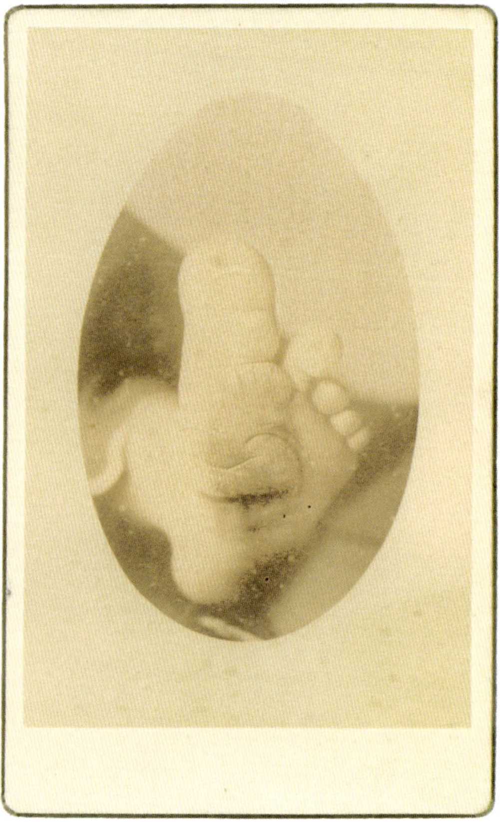

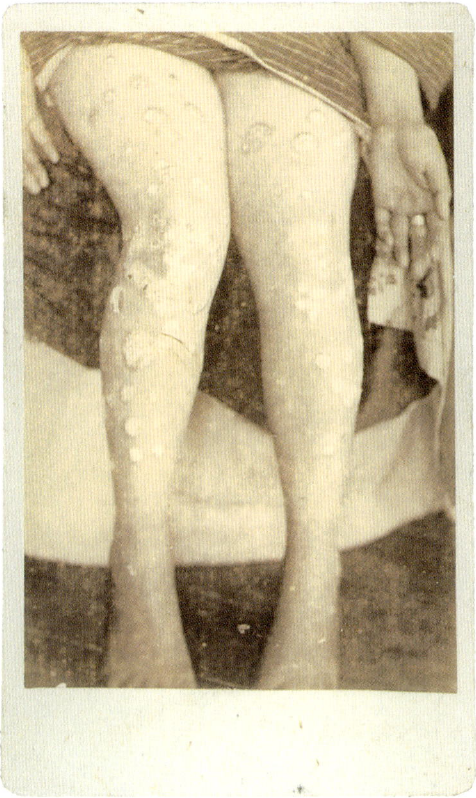

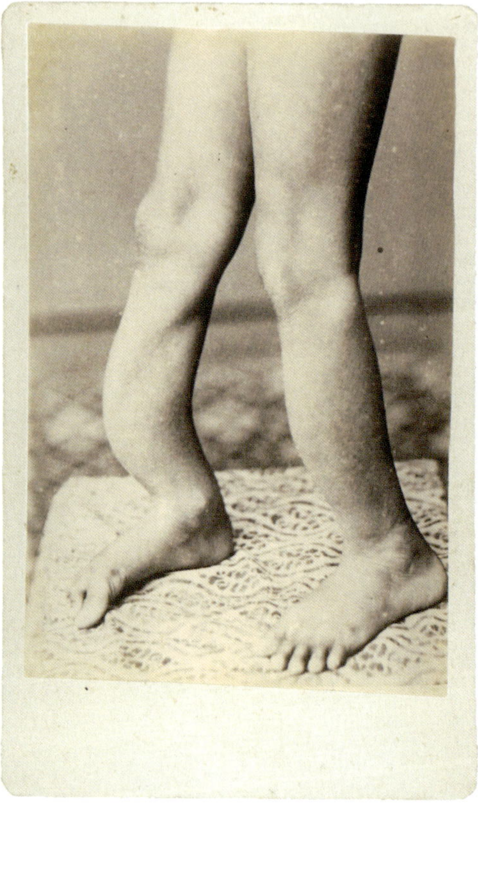

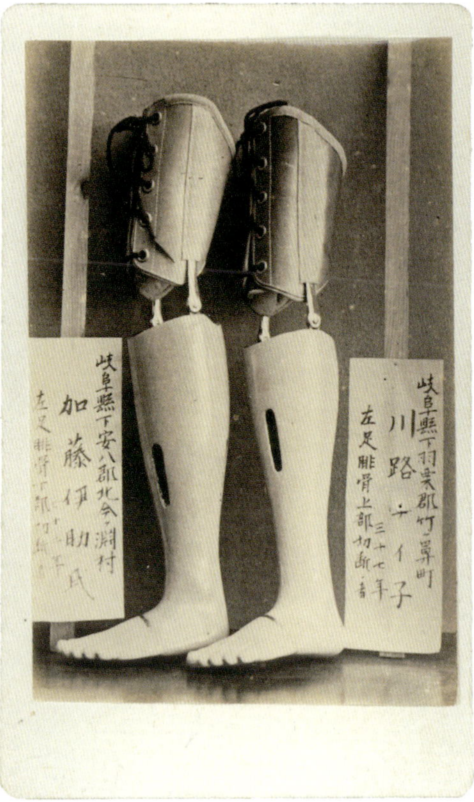
岐阜縣下安八郡北今ヶ淵村
加藤伊助氏
左足
岐阜縣下羽栗郡竹ヶ鼻町
川路ナイ子
左足腓骨上部切断者
三十七年

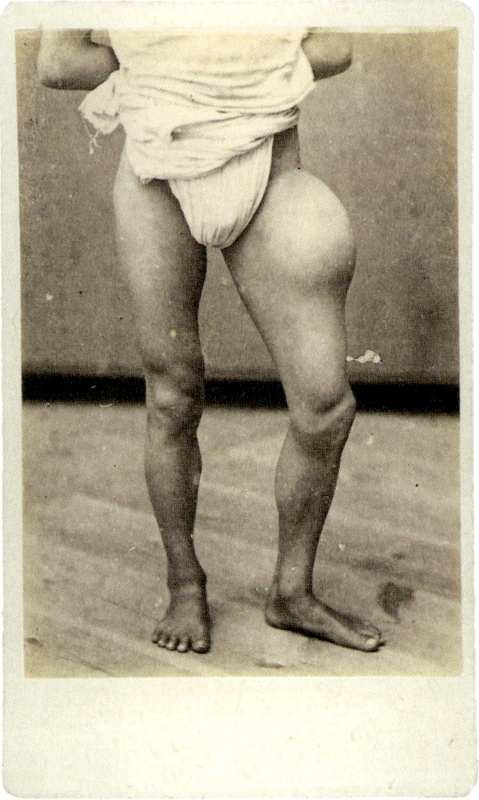

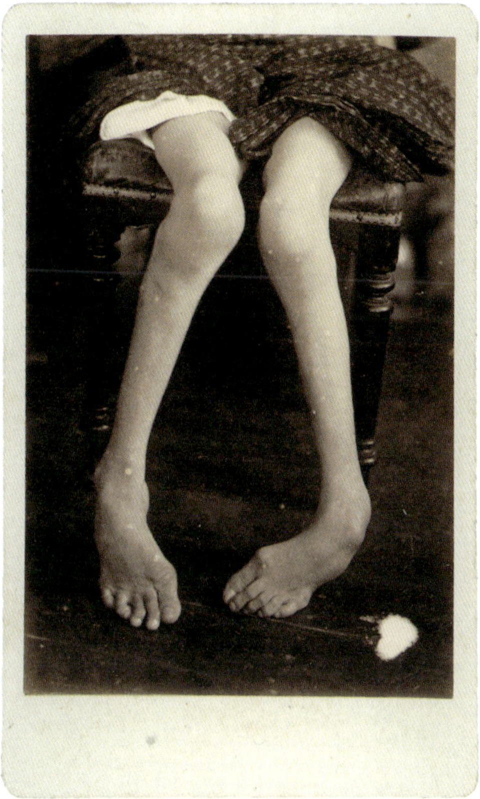

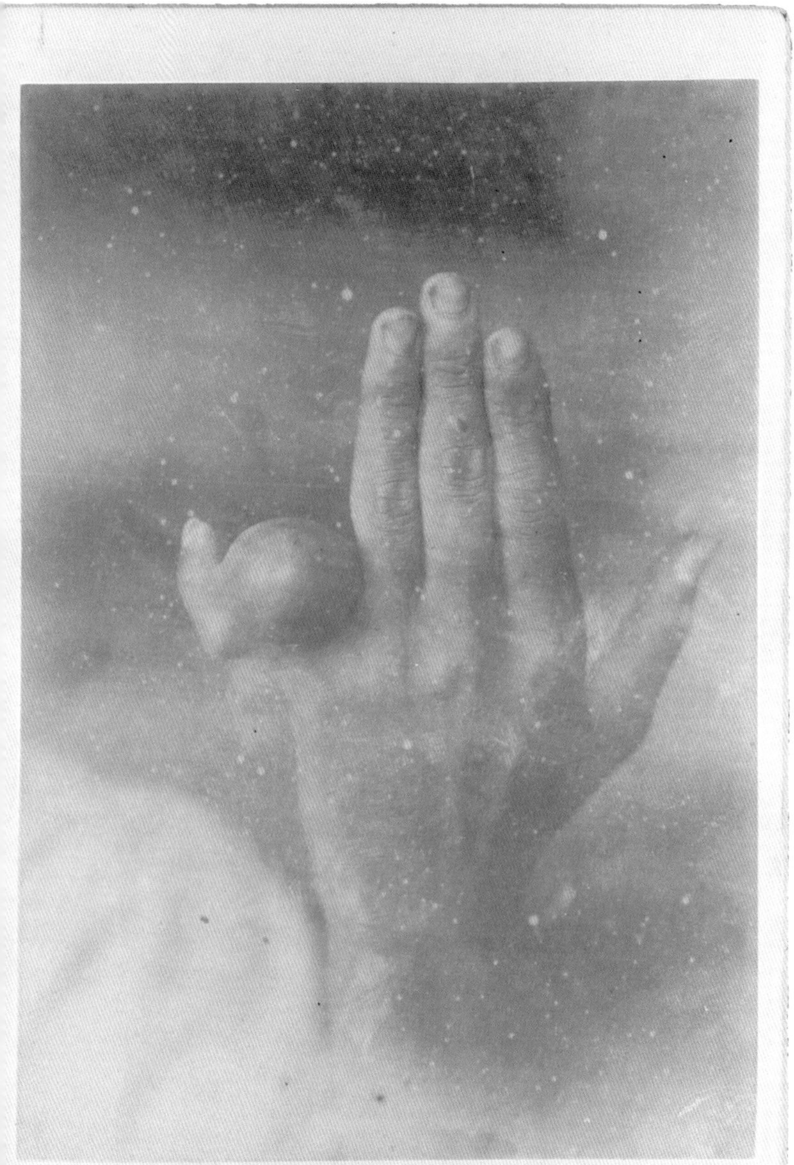

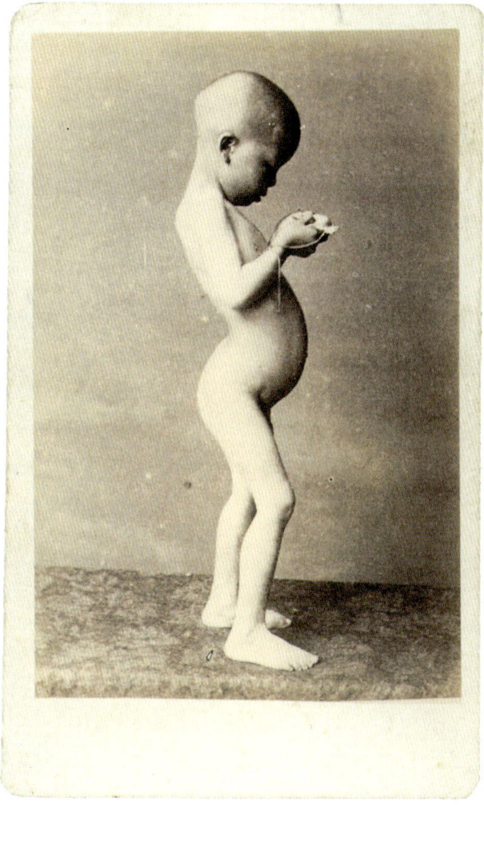

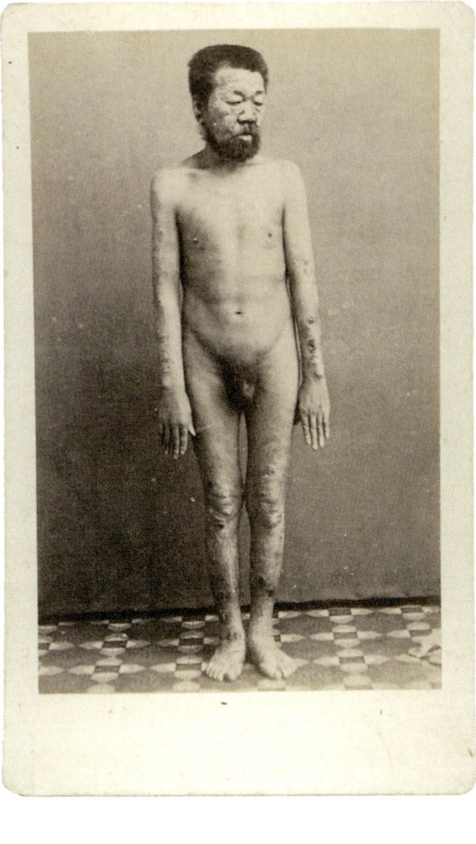

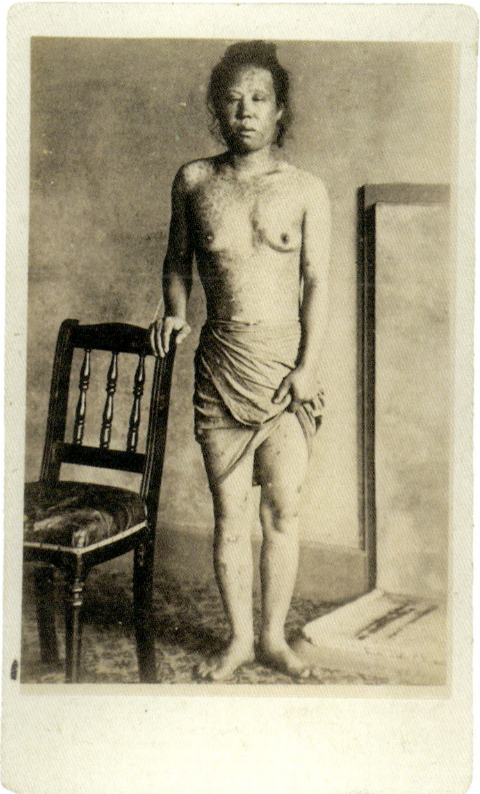

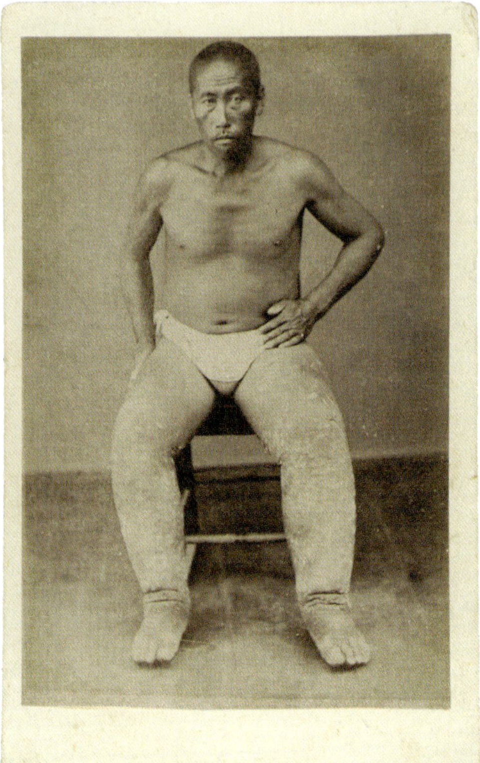

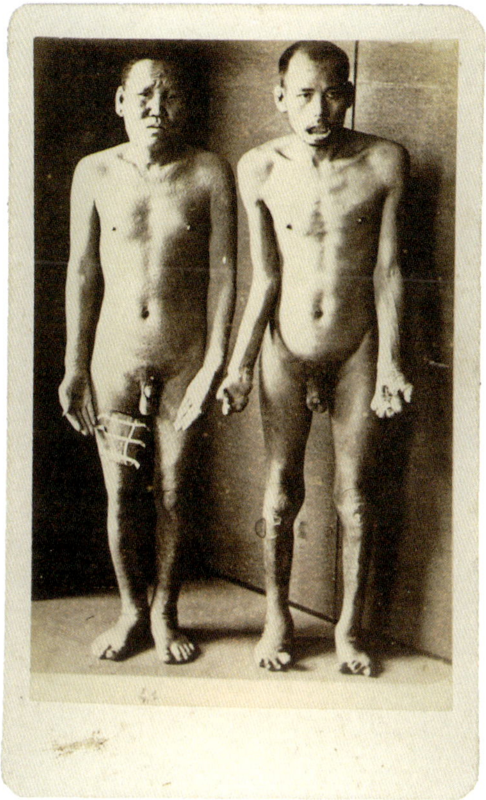

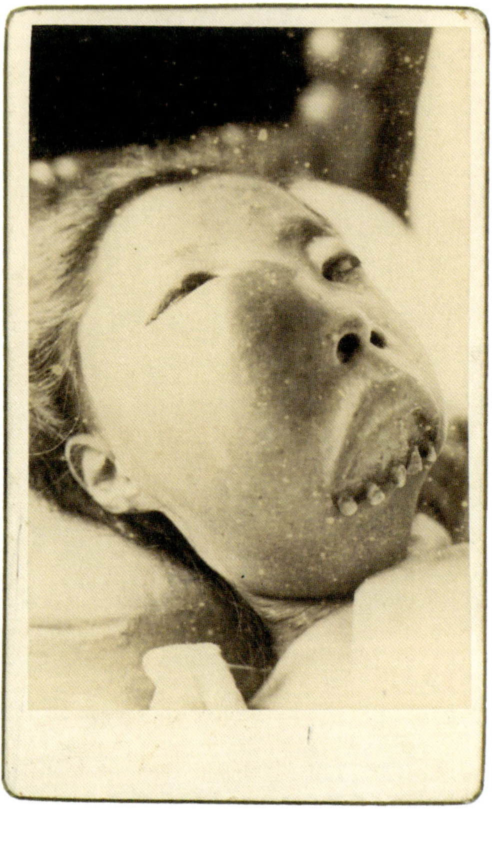

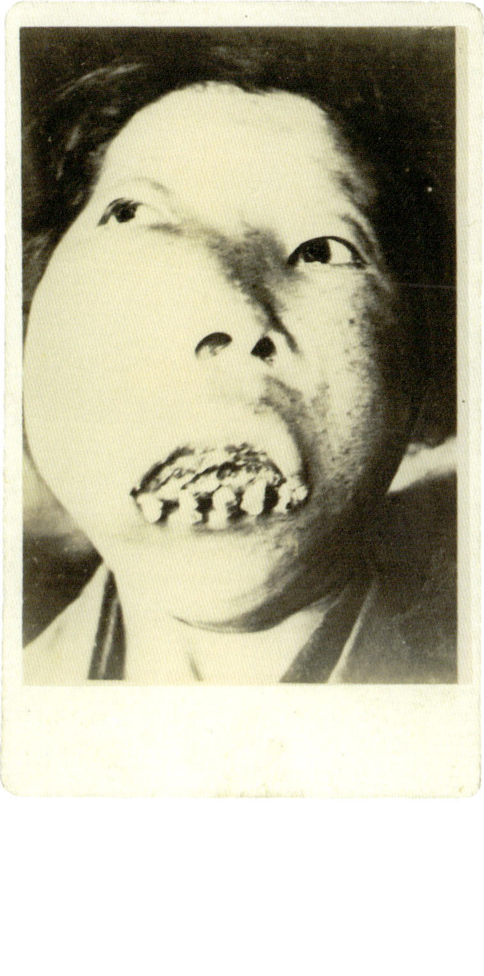

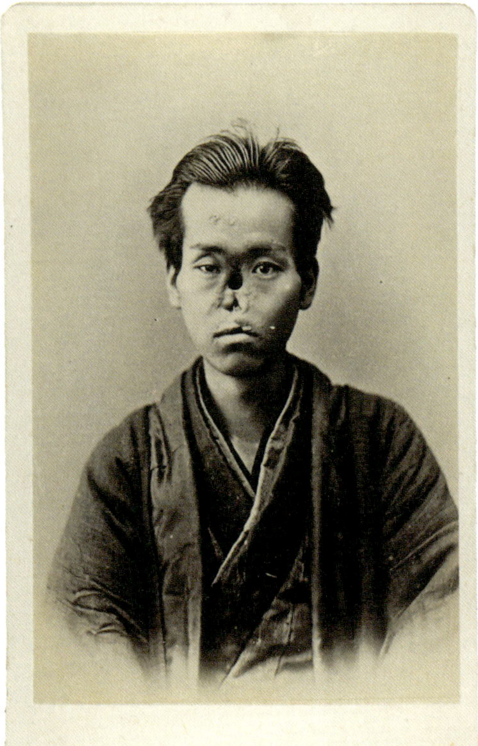

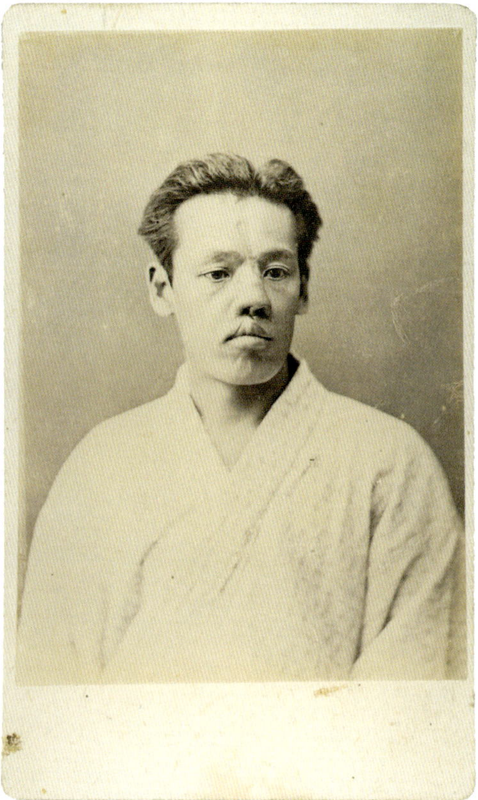

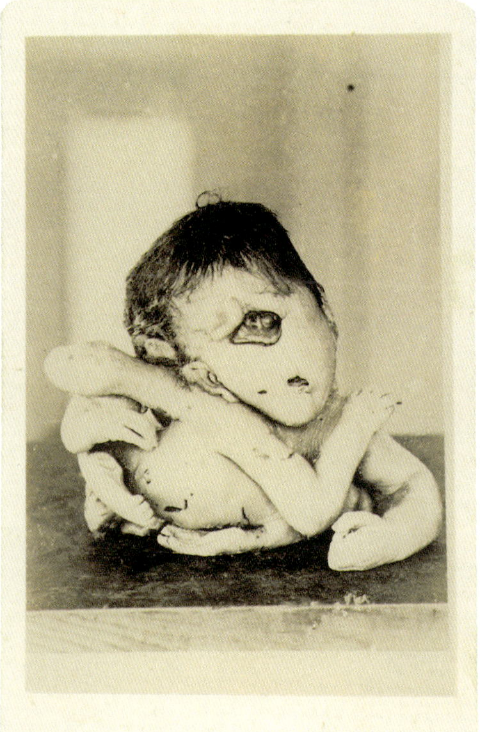

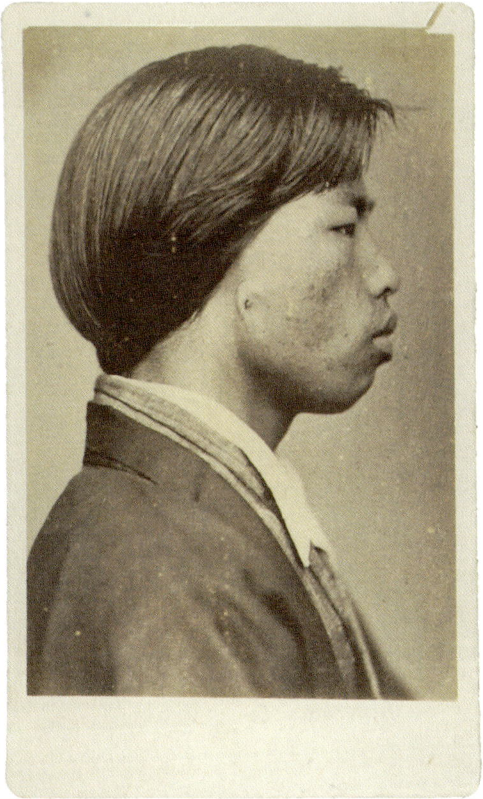

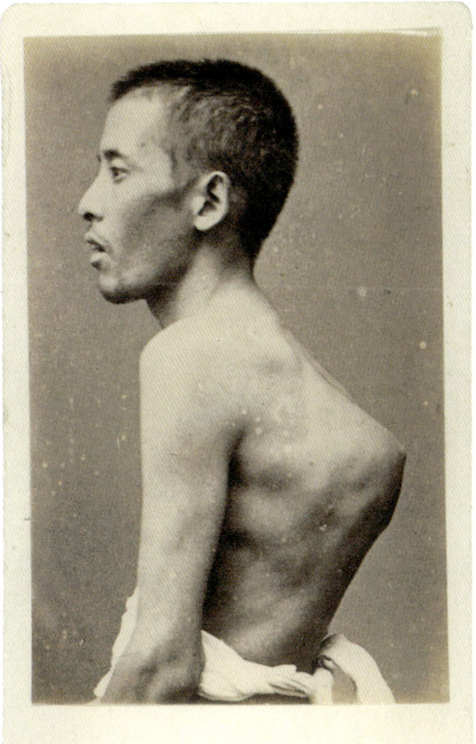

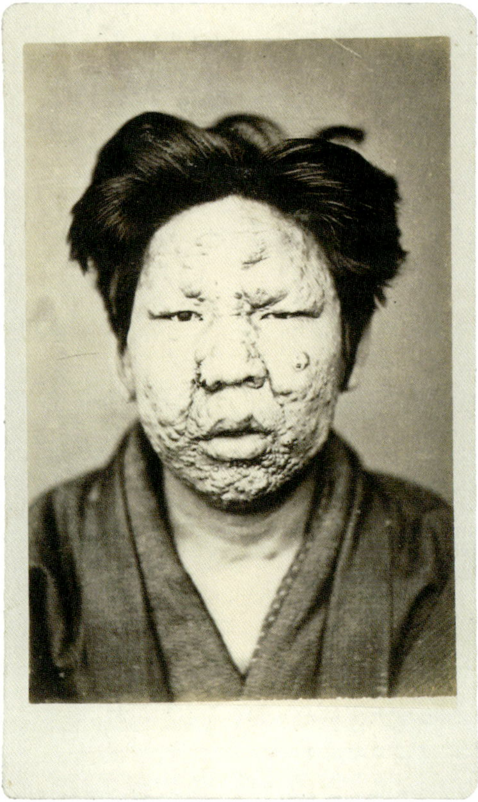

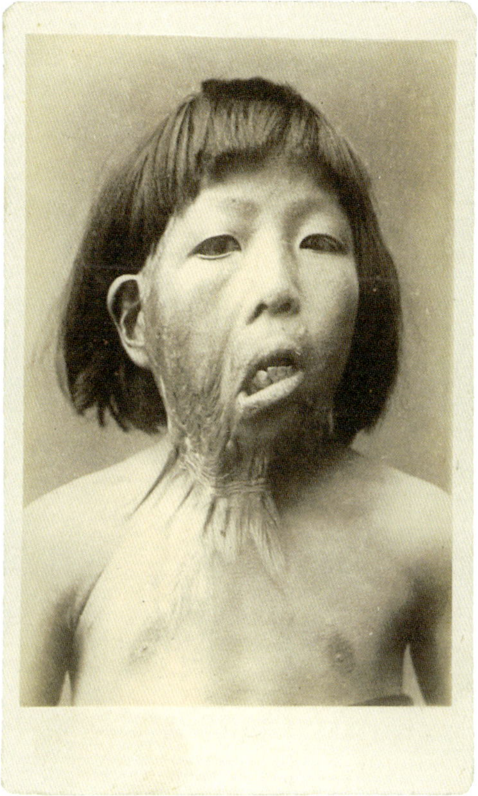

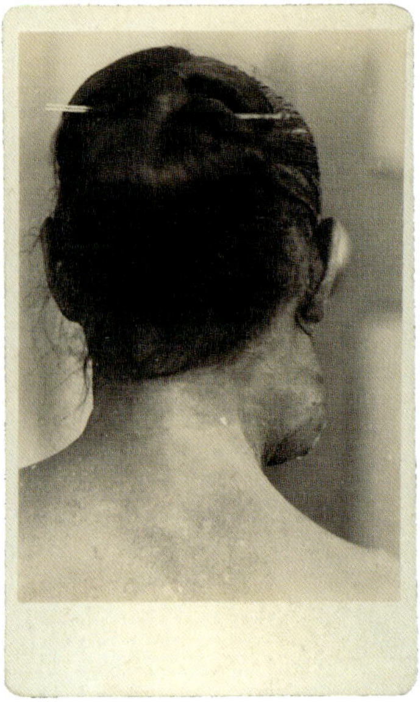

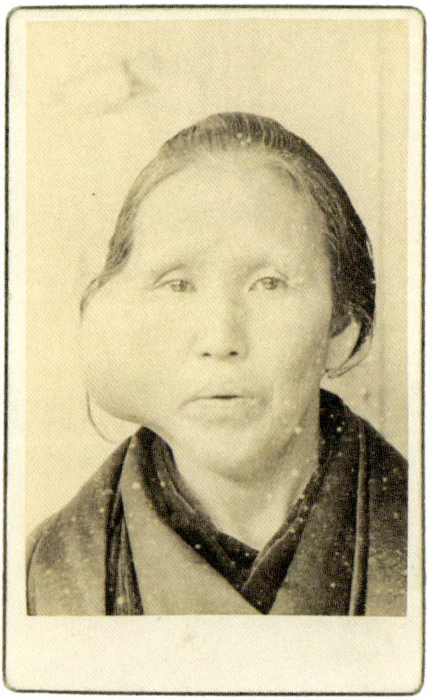

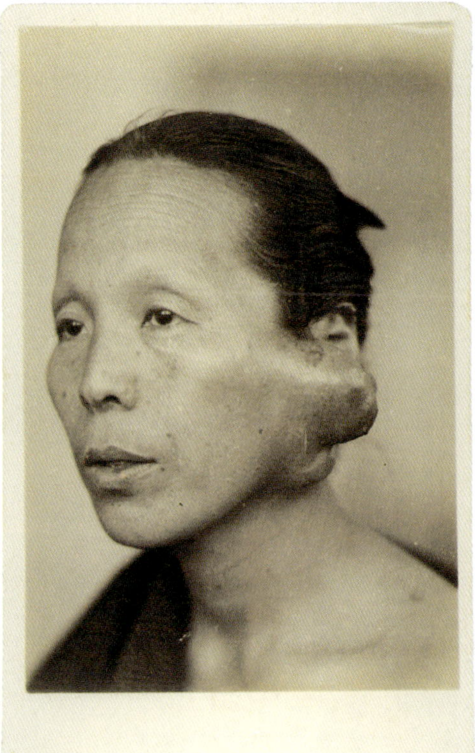

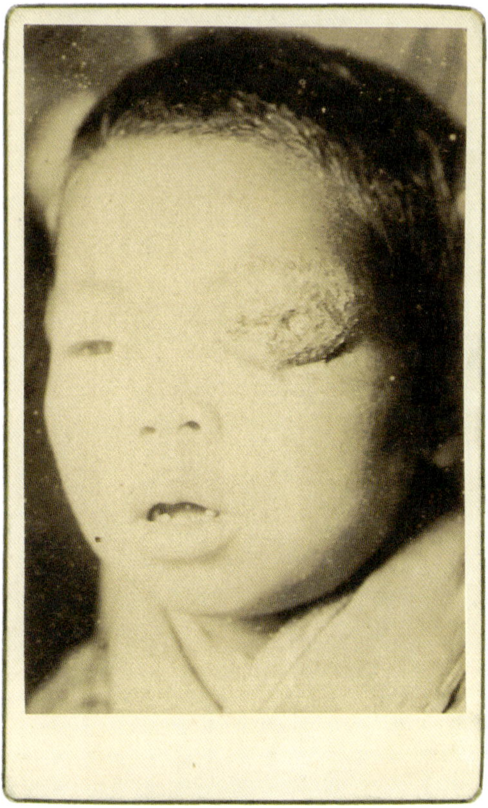

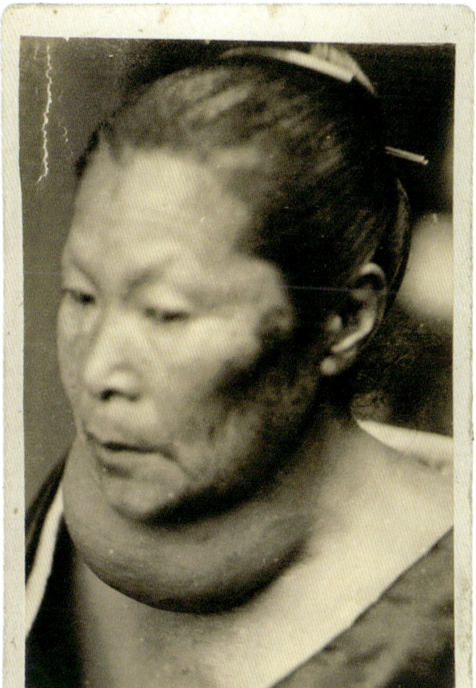

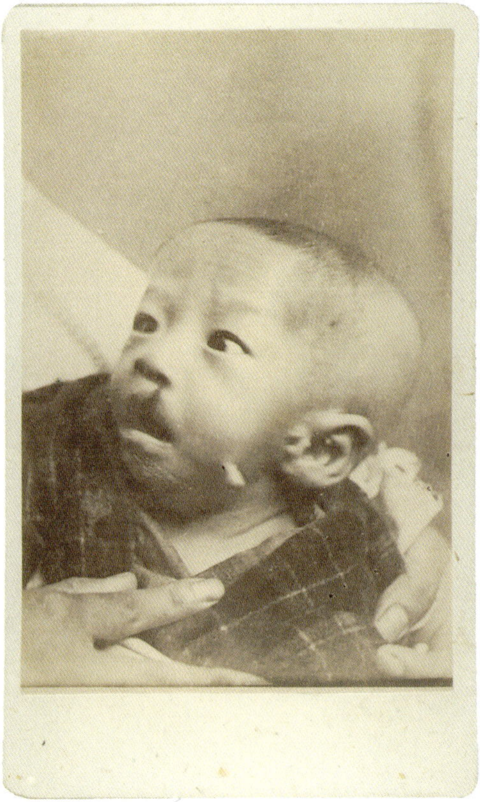

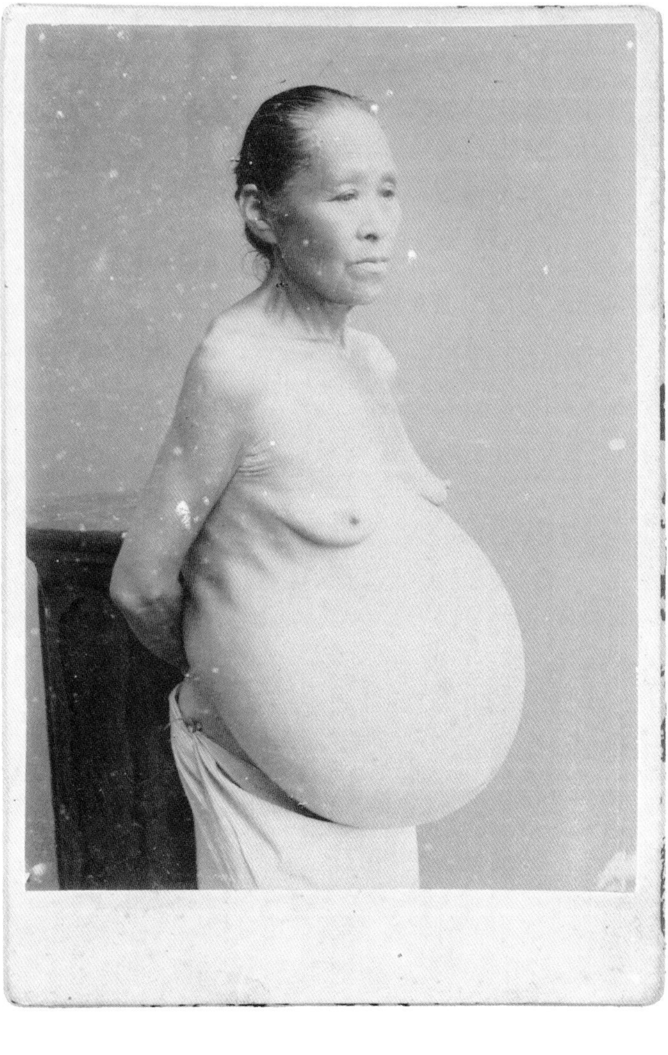

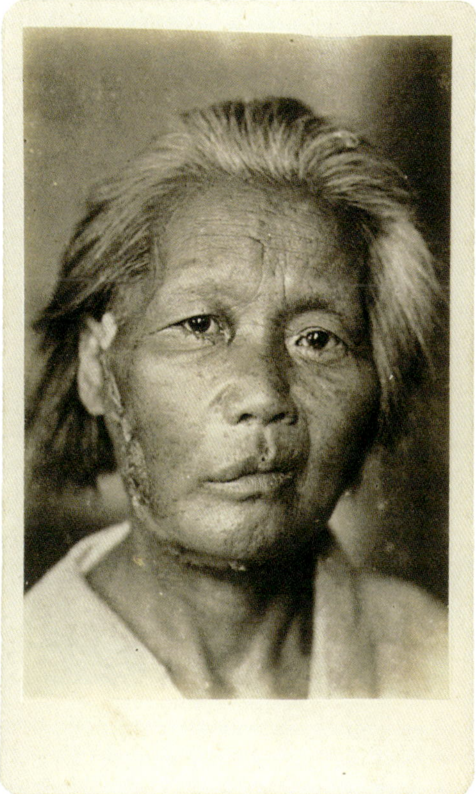

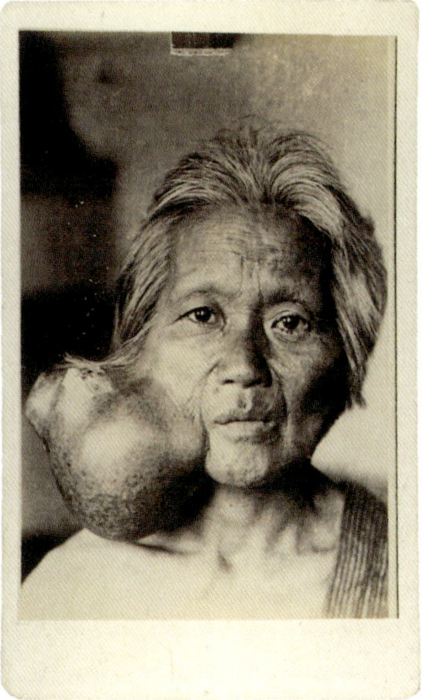

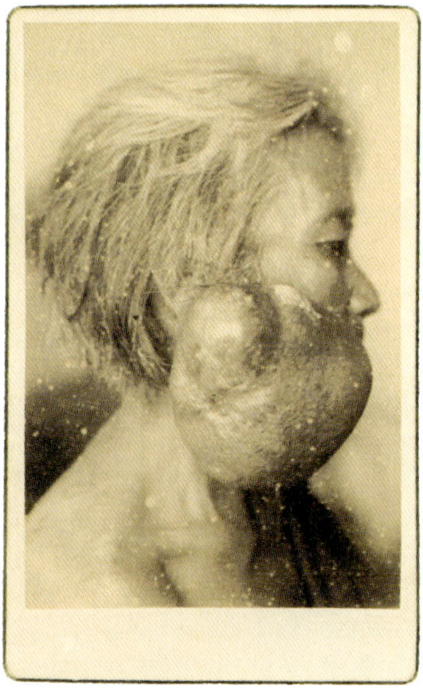

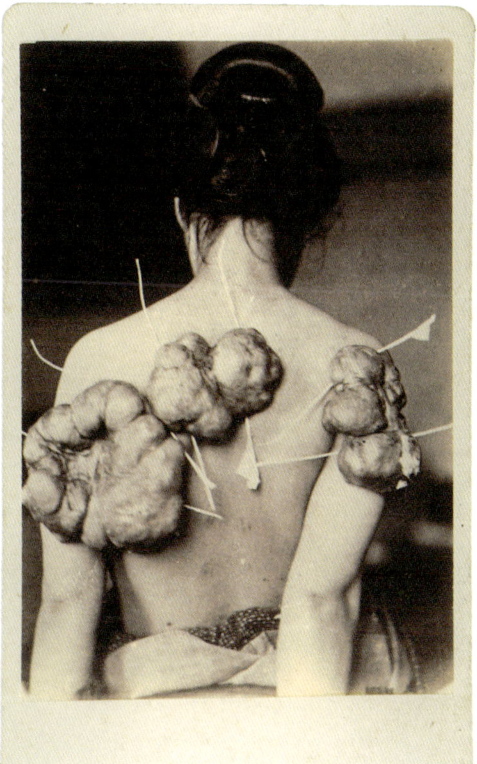

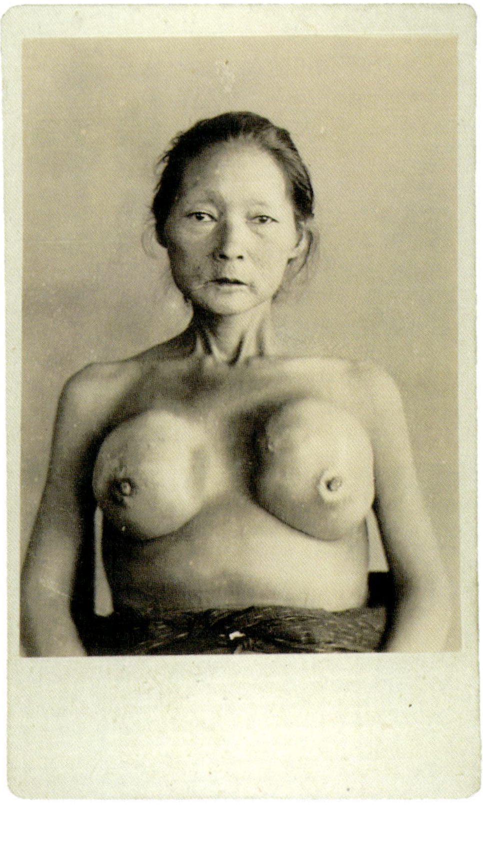

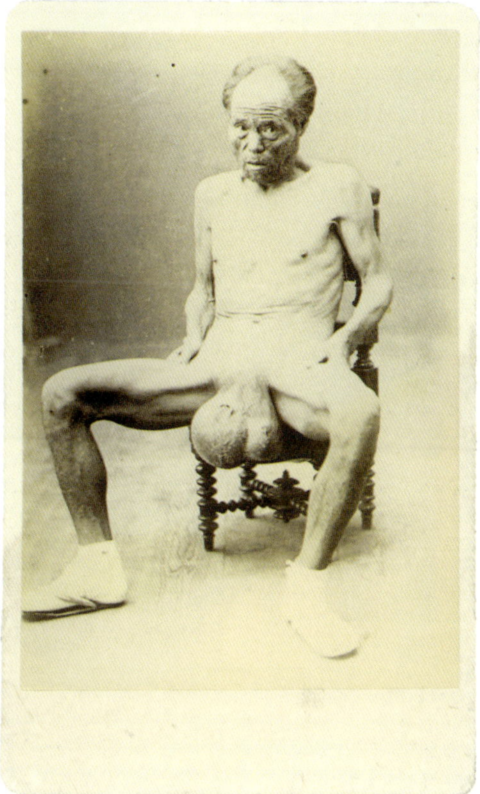

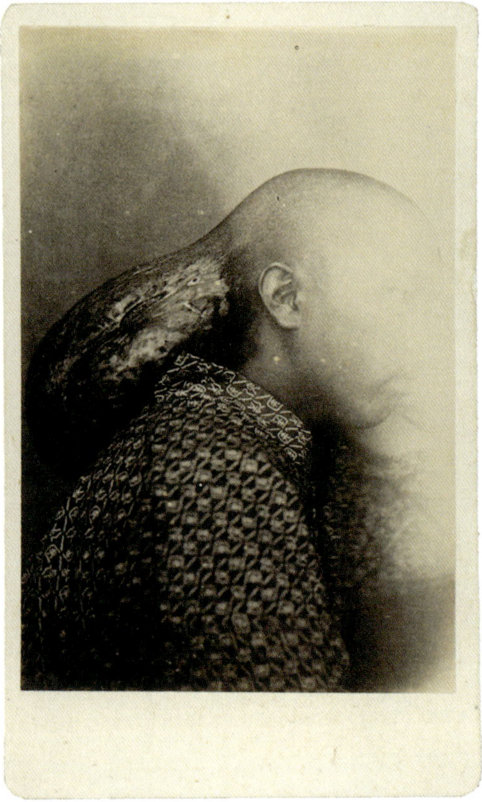

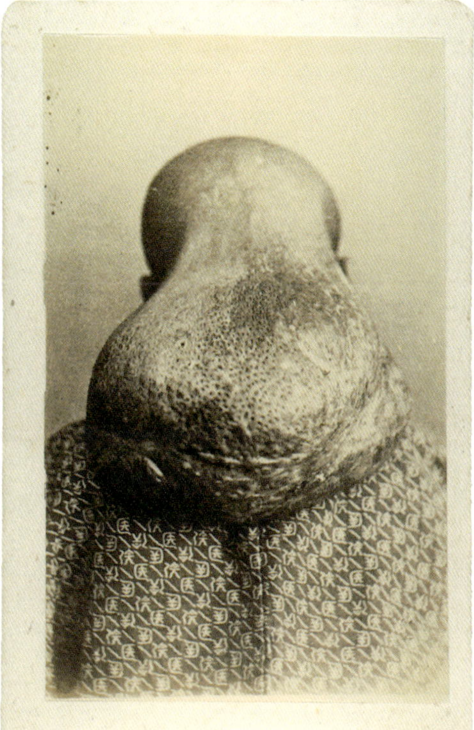

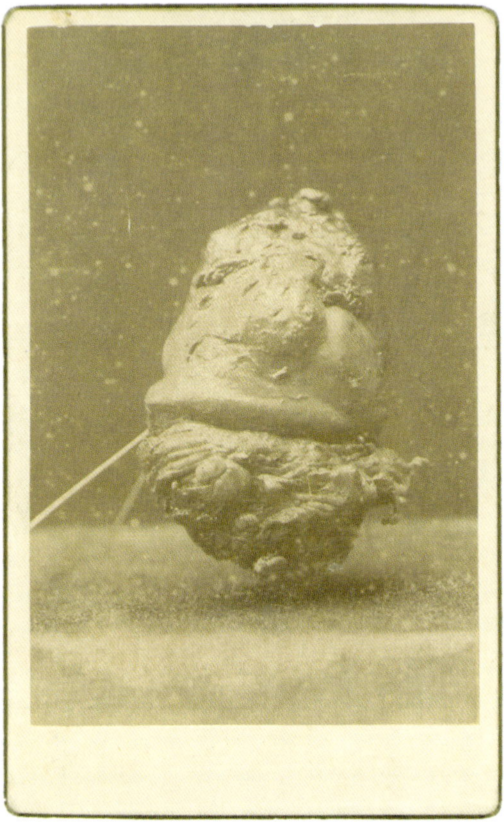

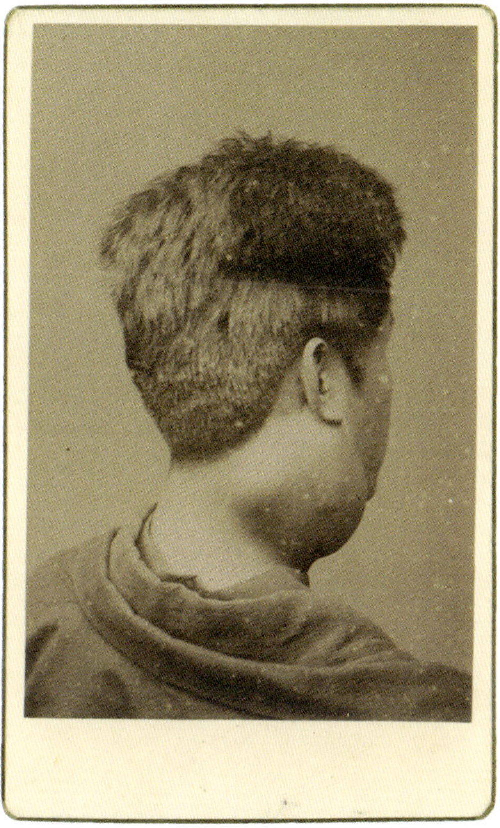

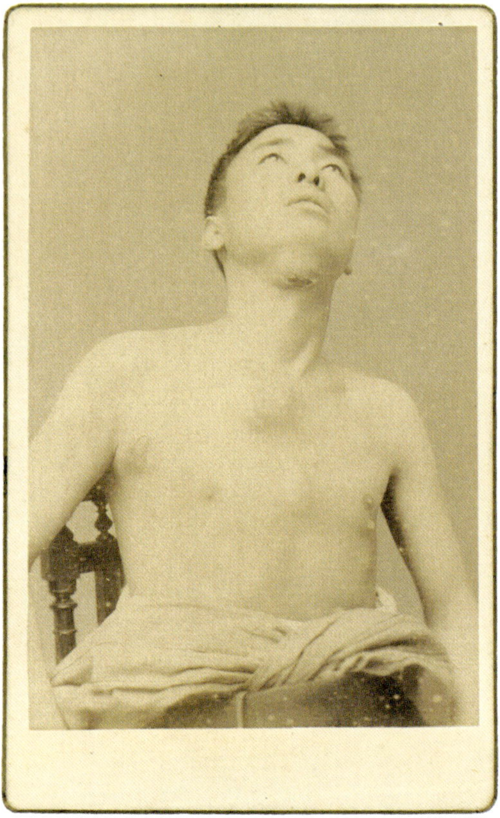

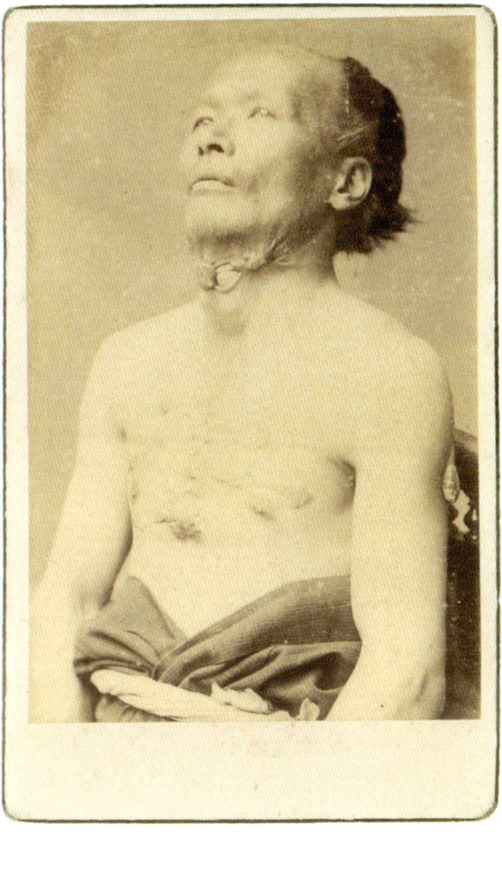

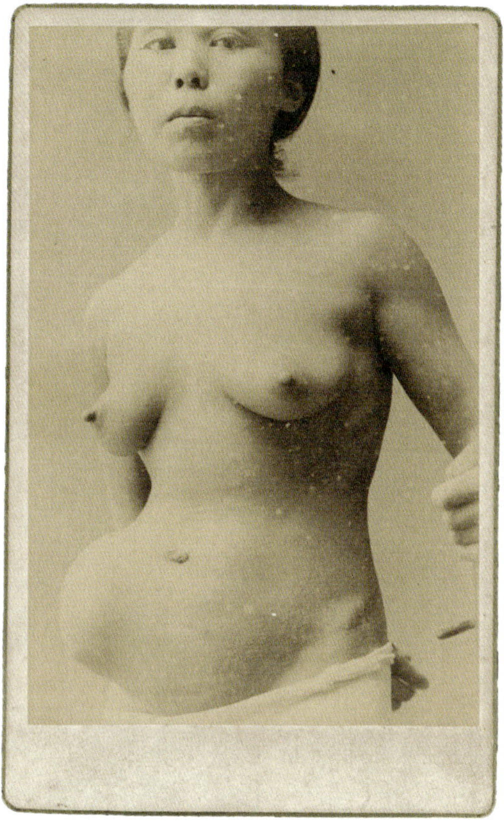

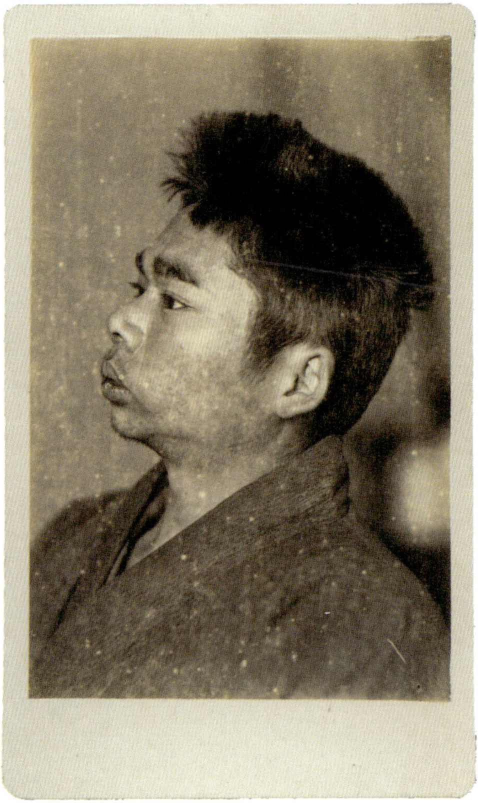

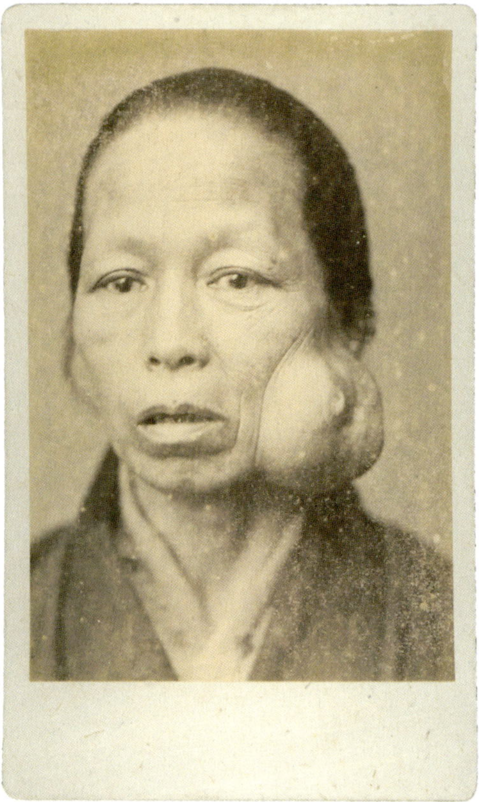

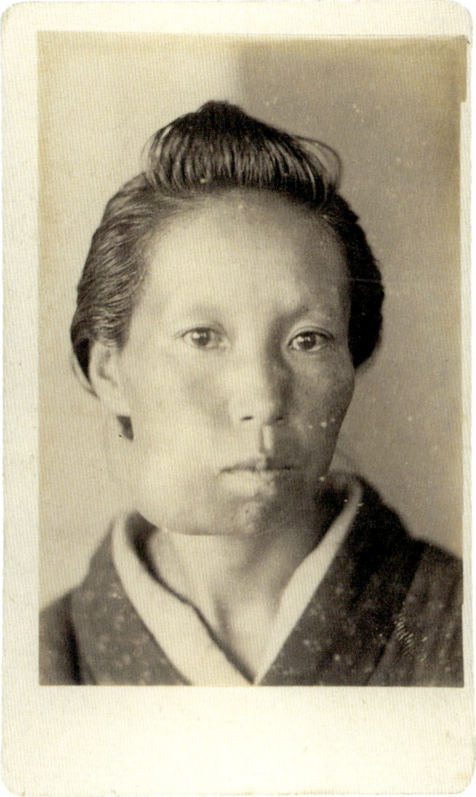

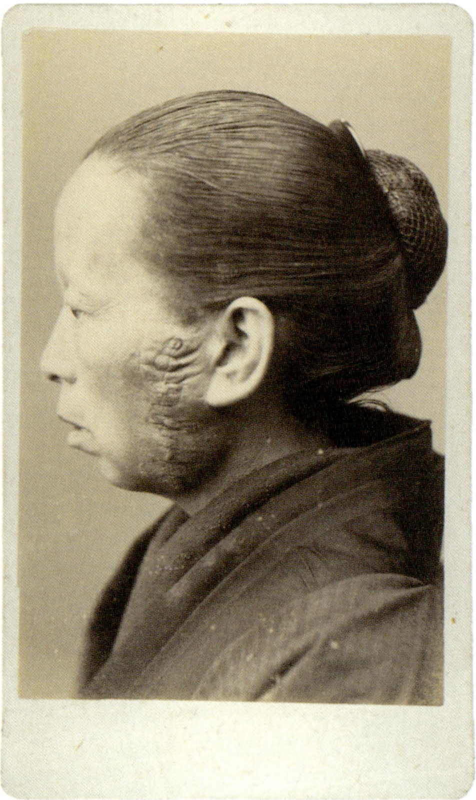

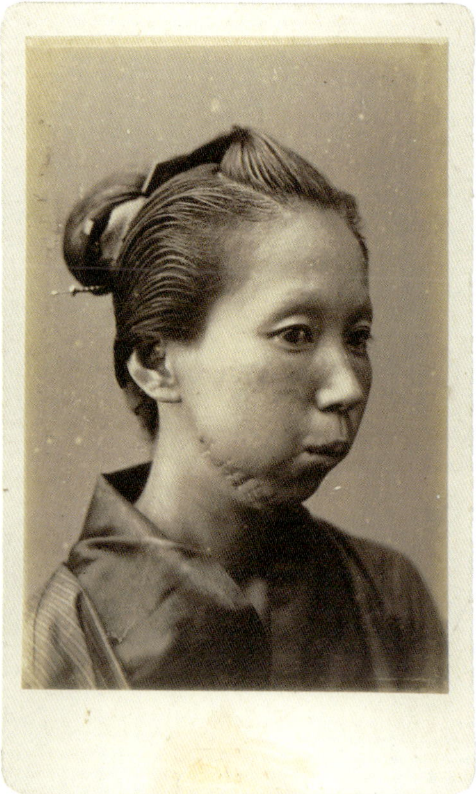

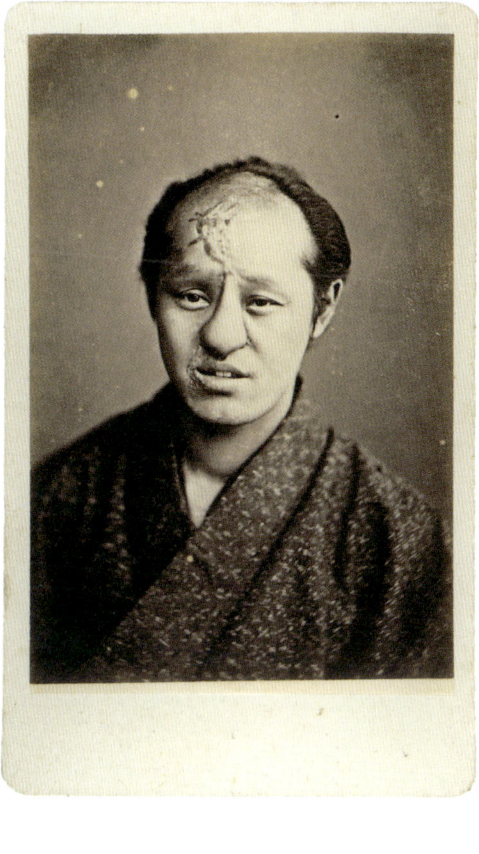

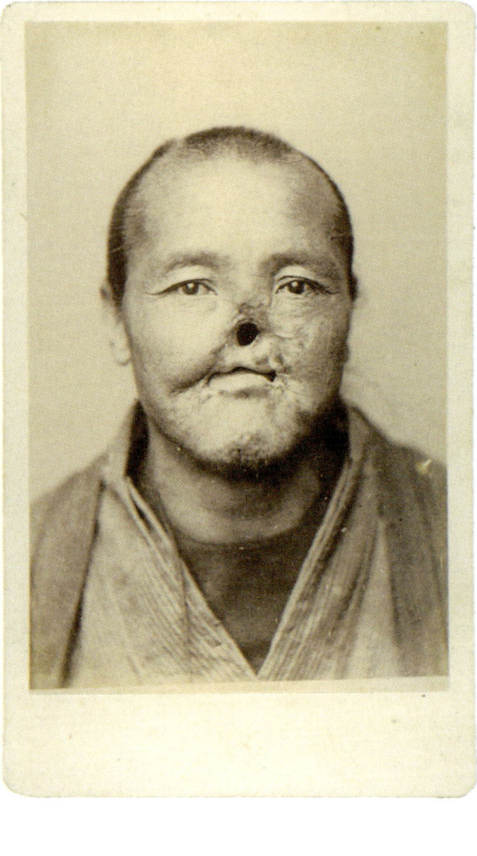

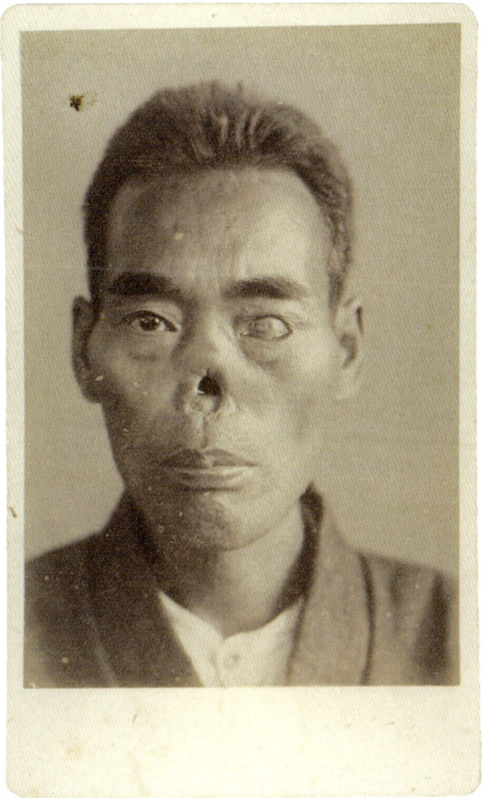

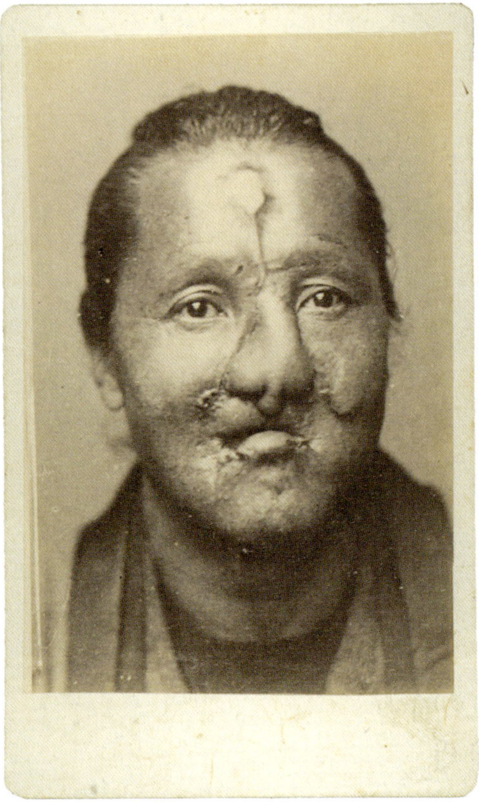

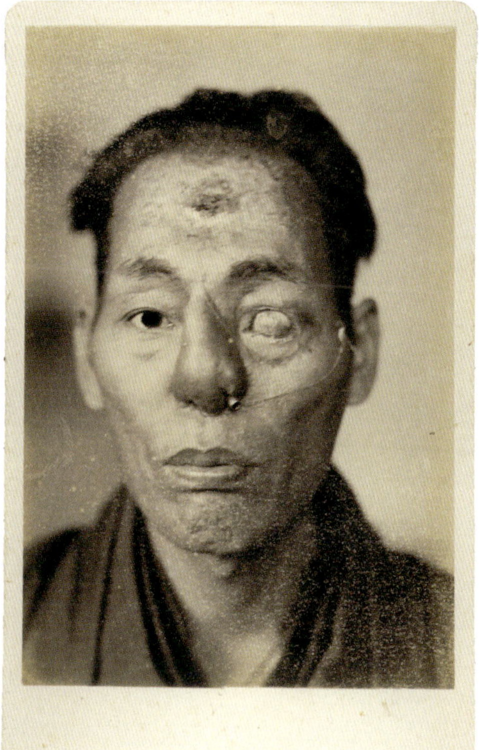

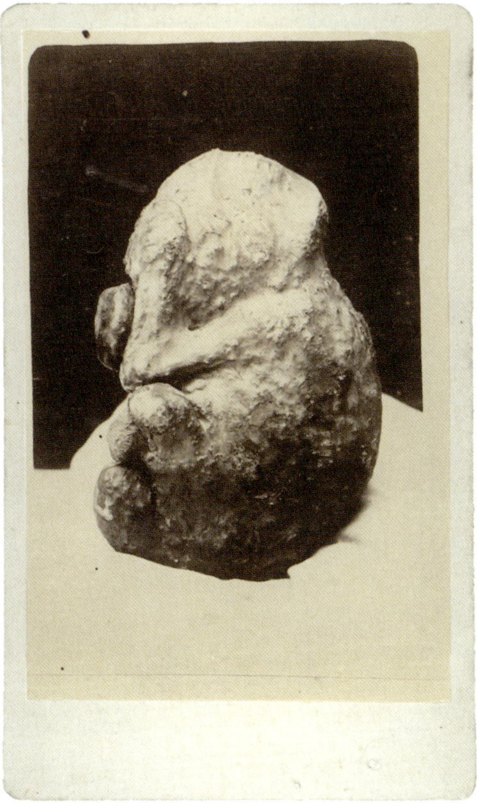

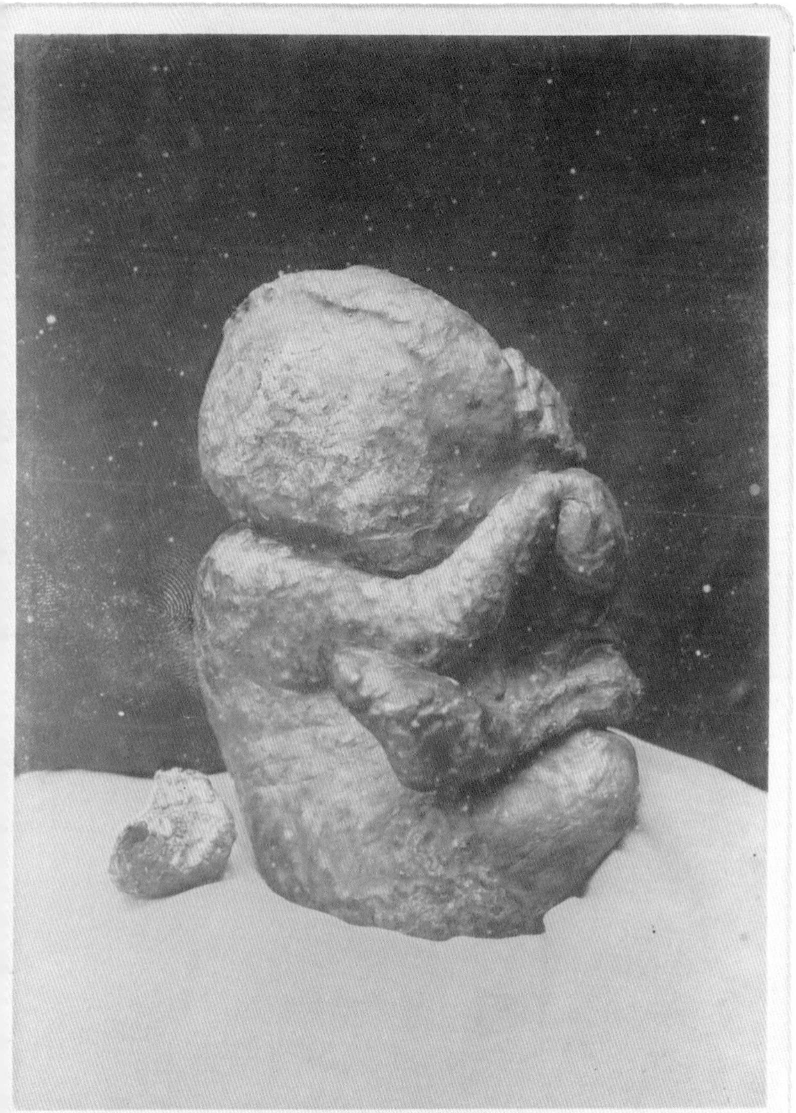

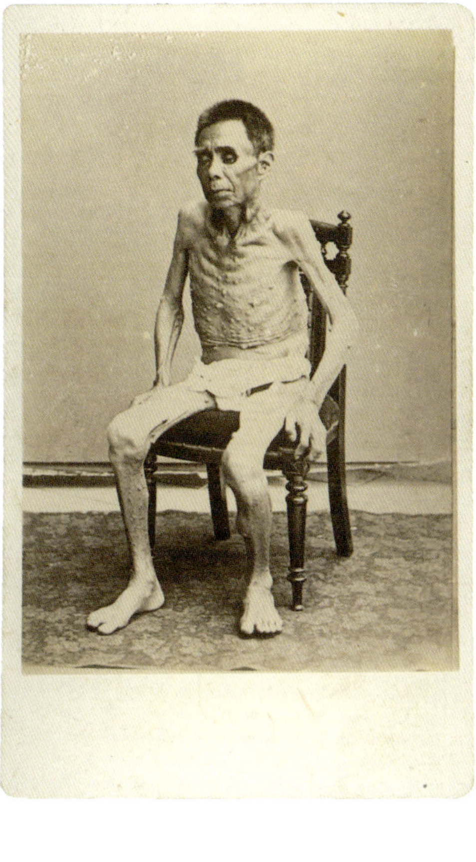

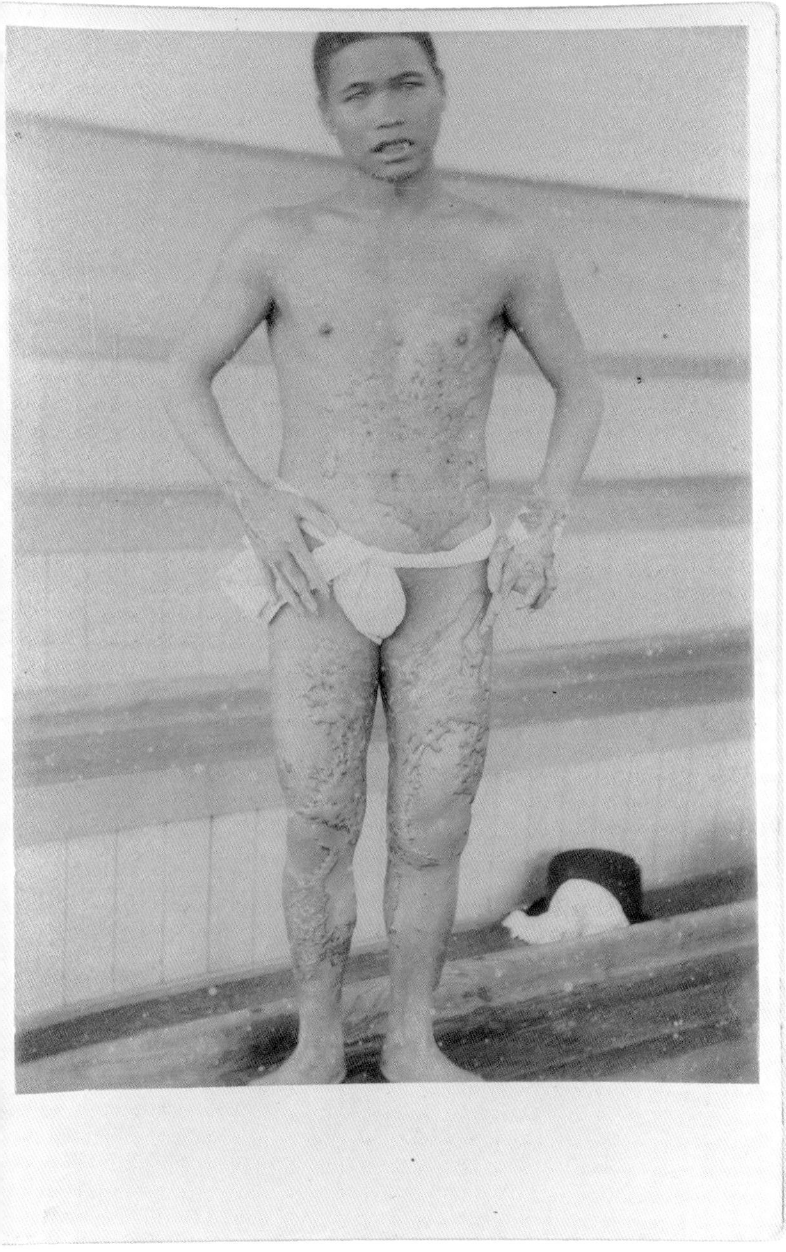

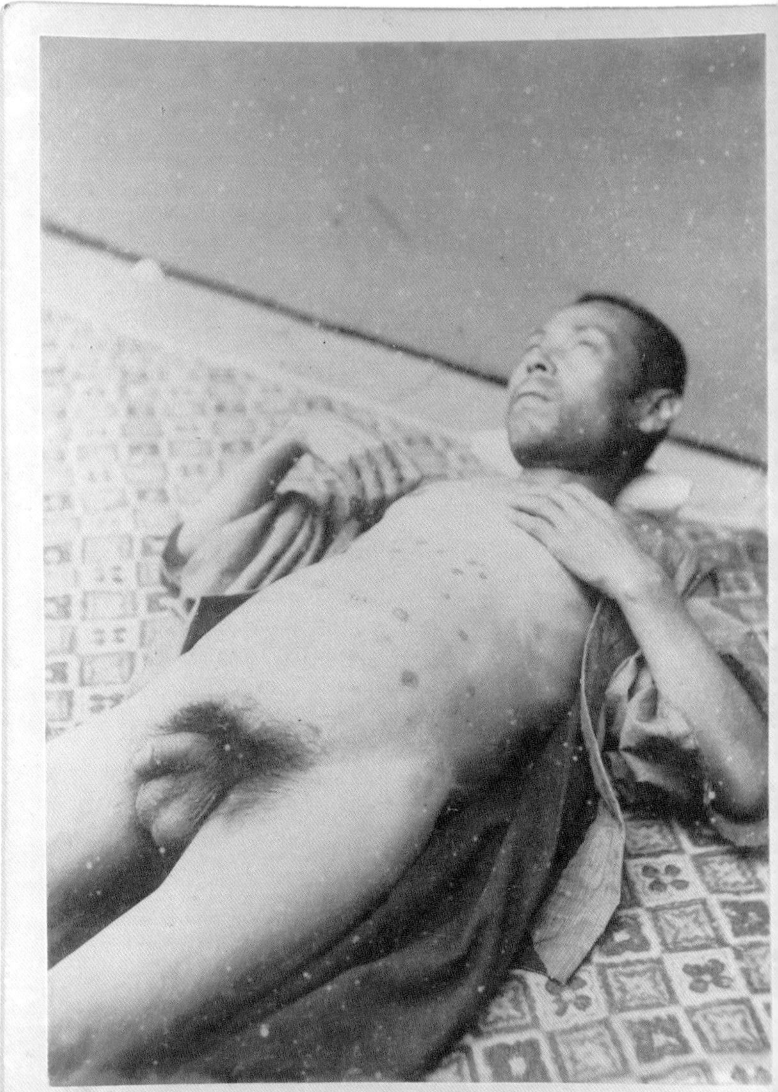

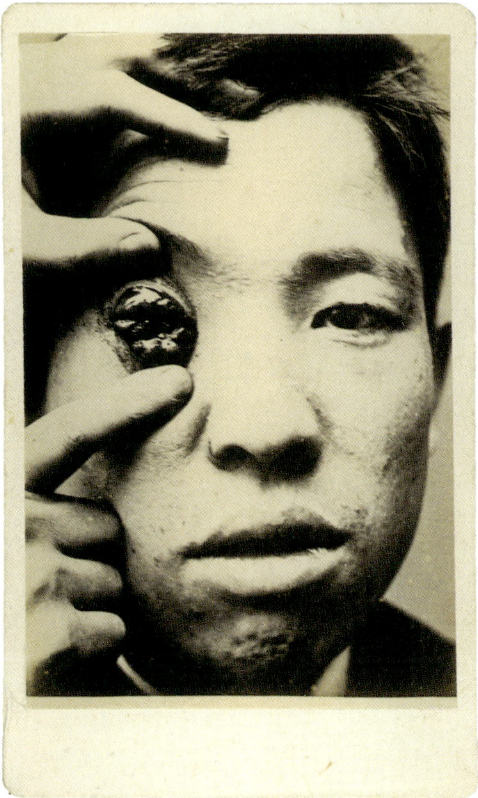

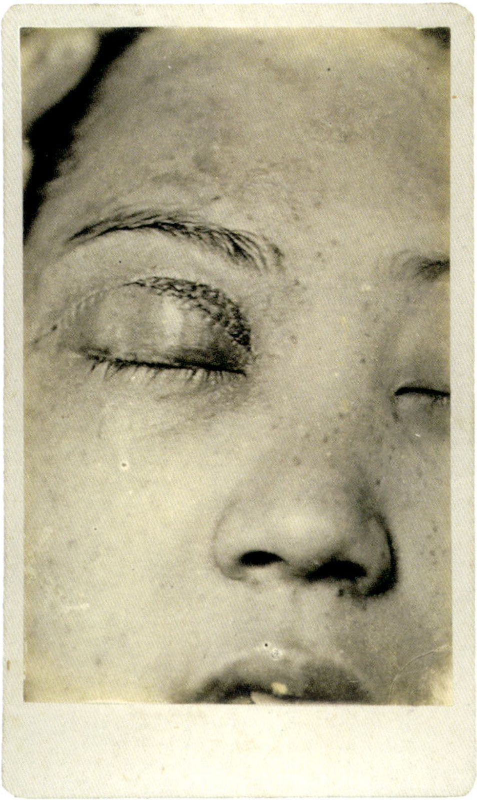

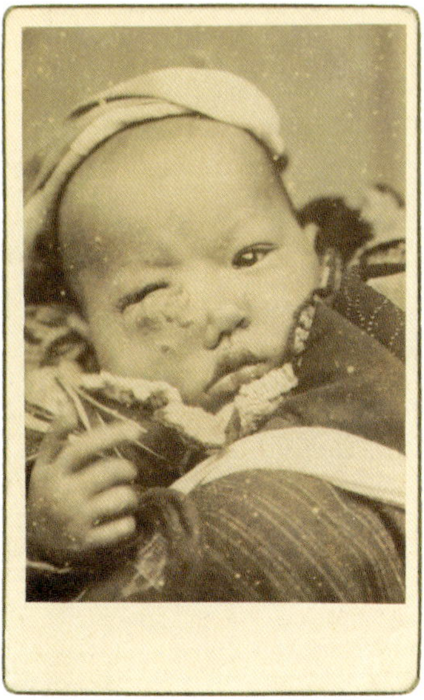

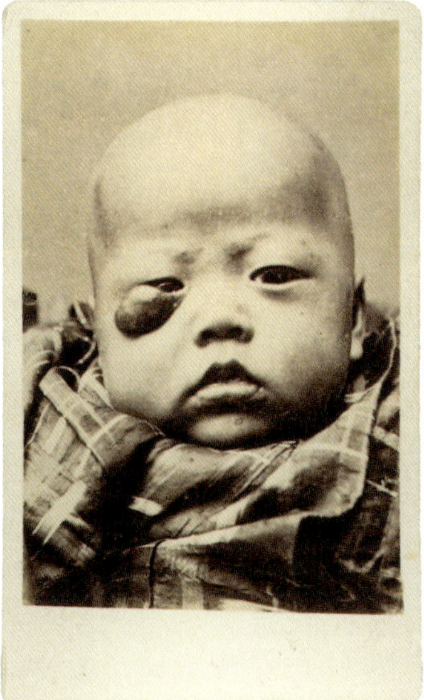

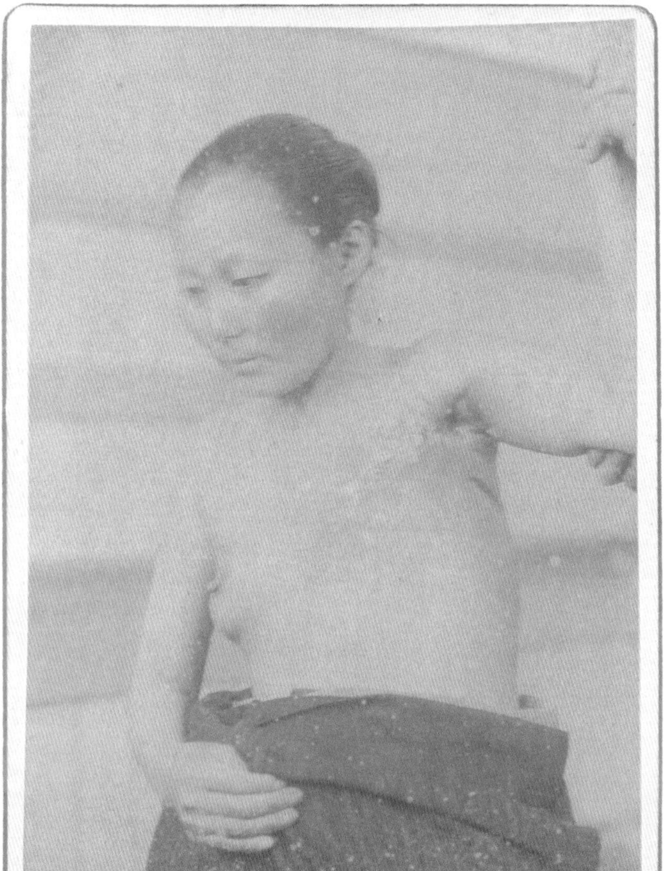

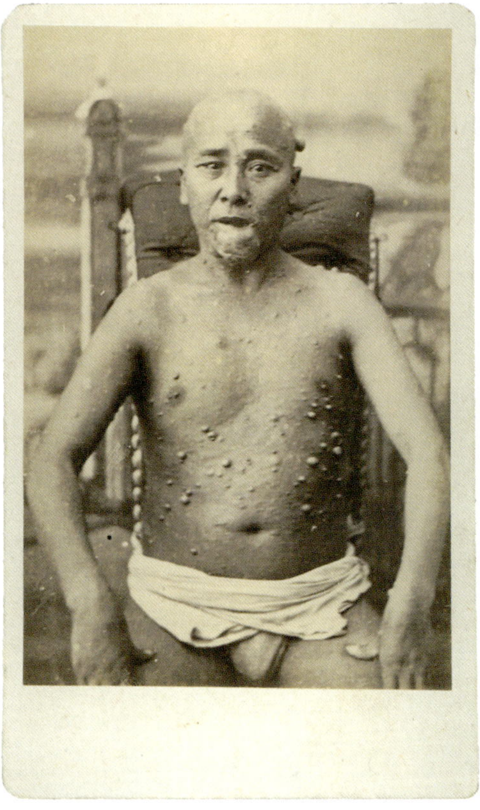

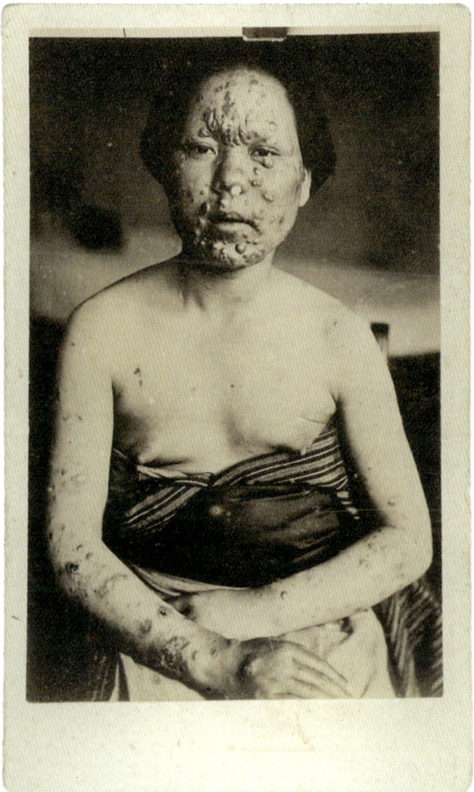

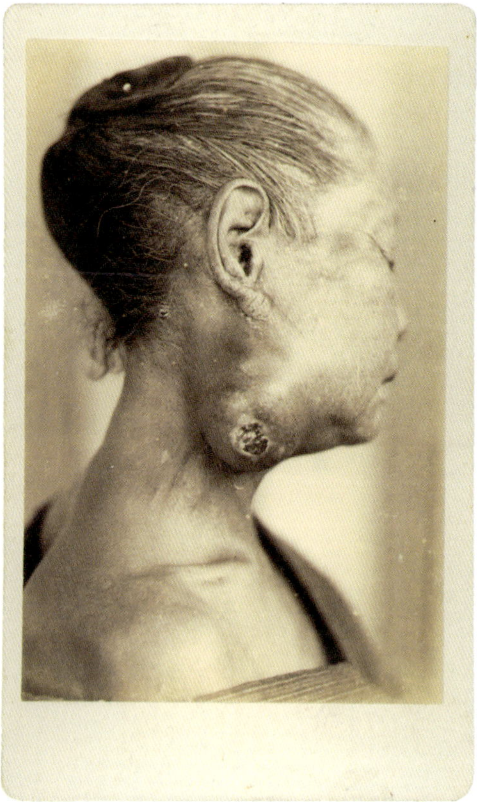

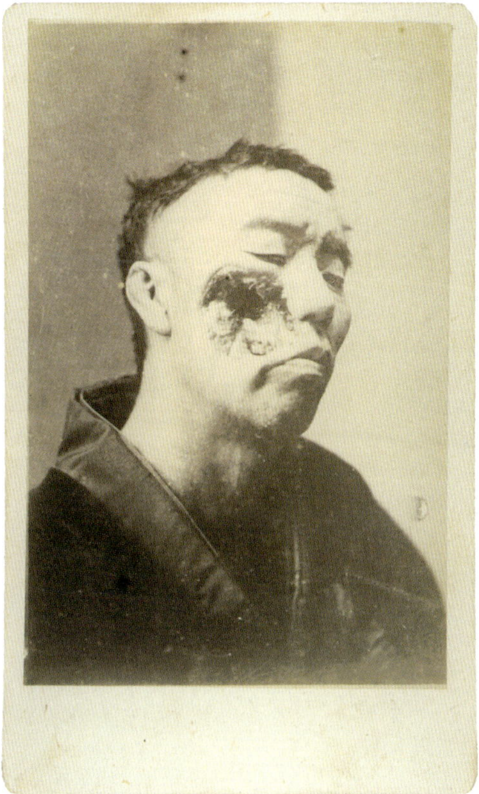

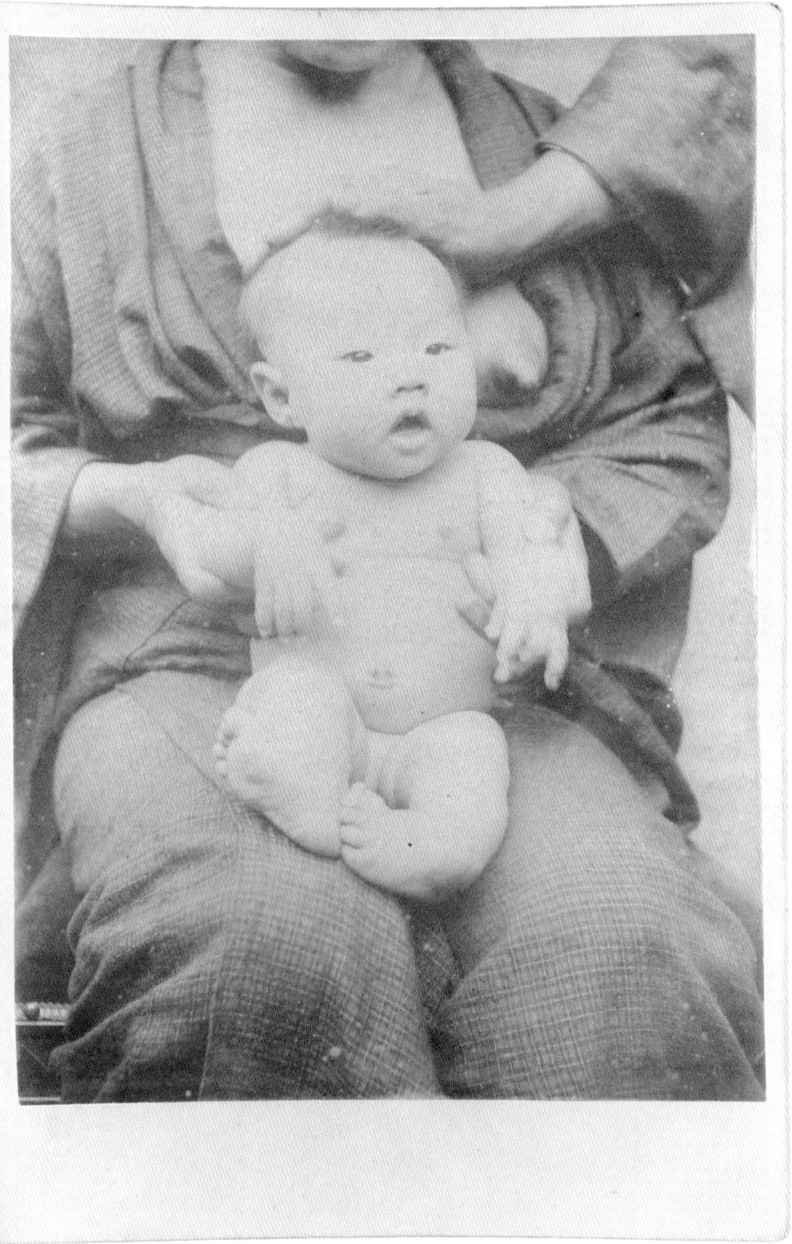

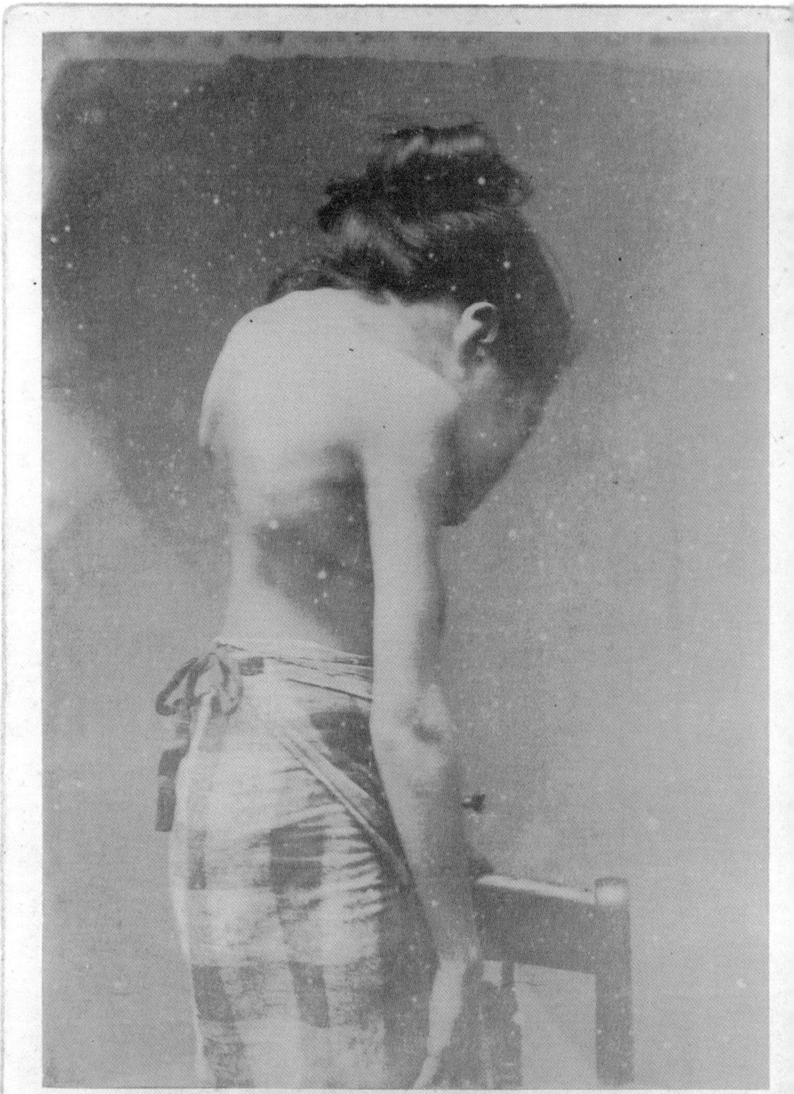

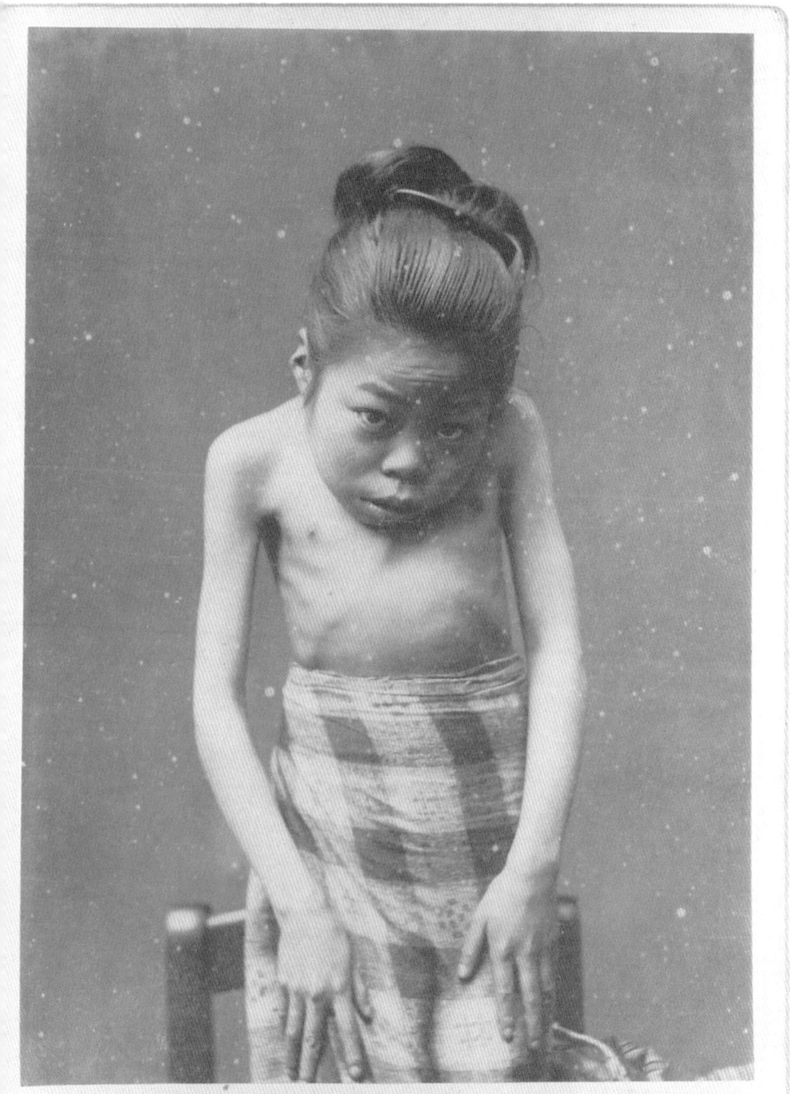

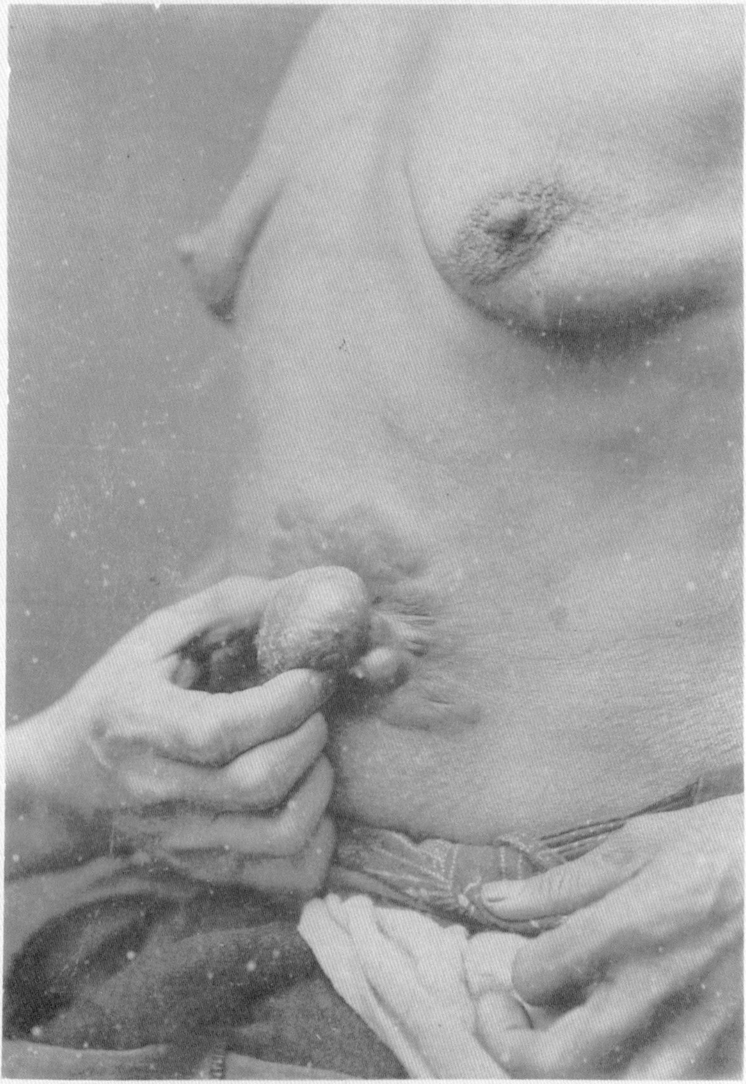

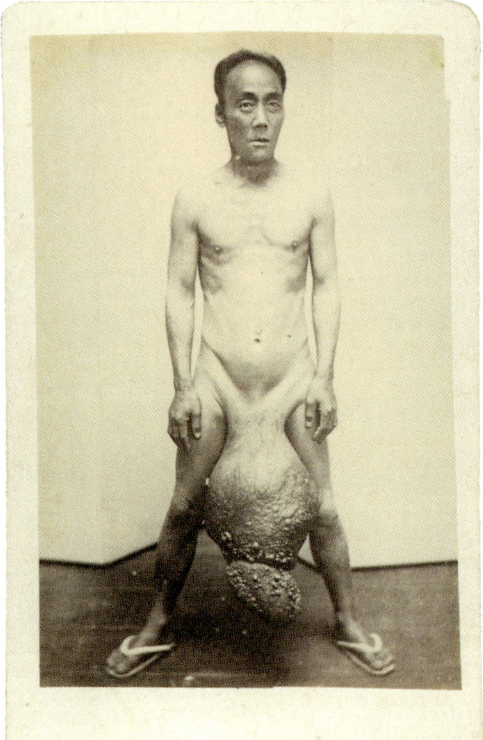

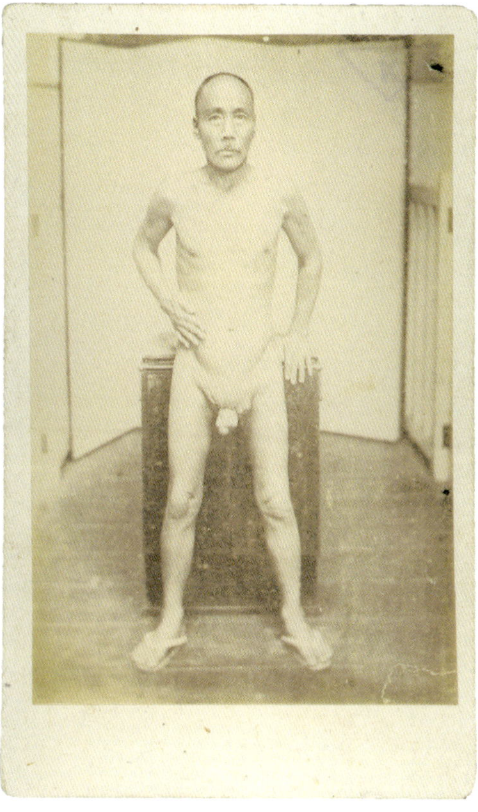

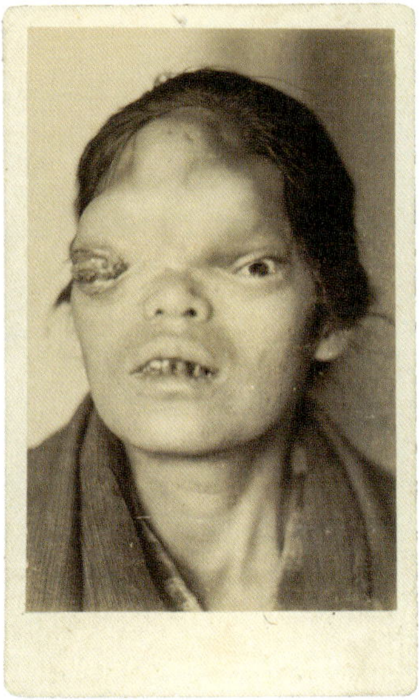

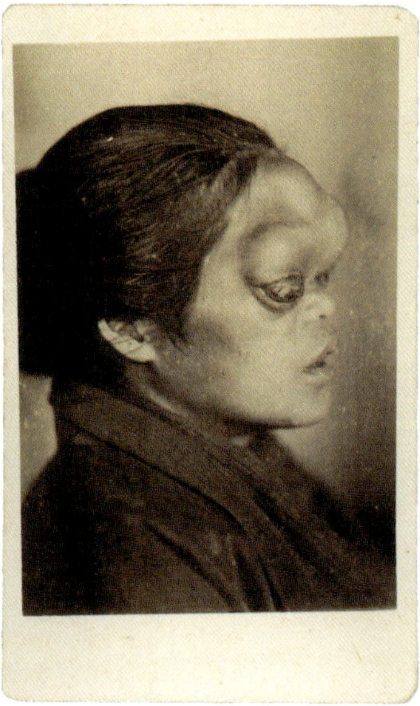

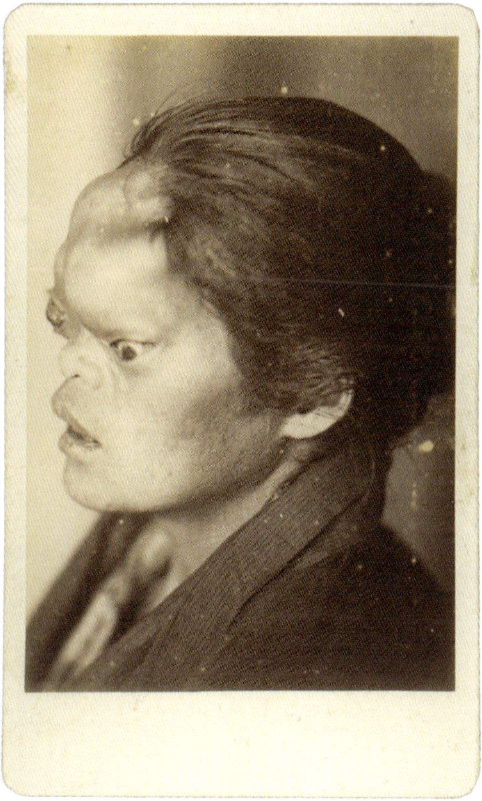

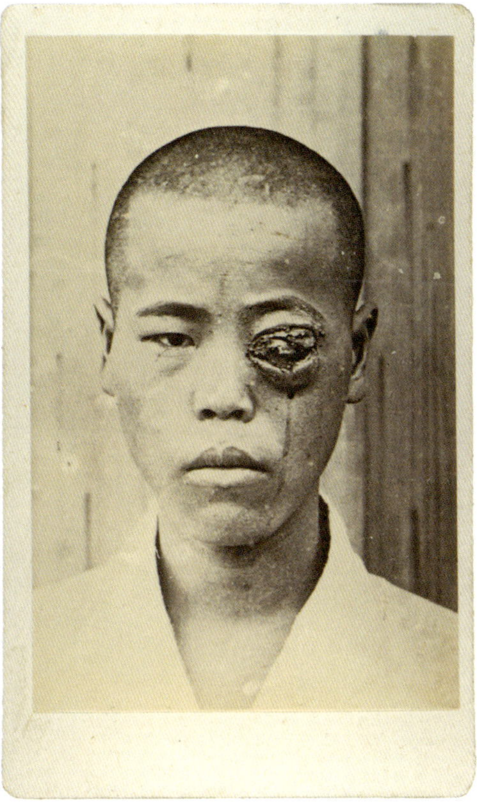

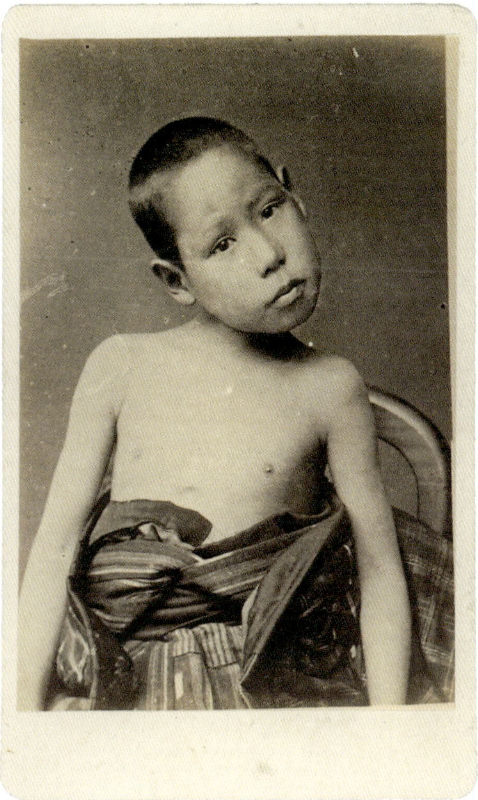

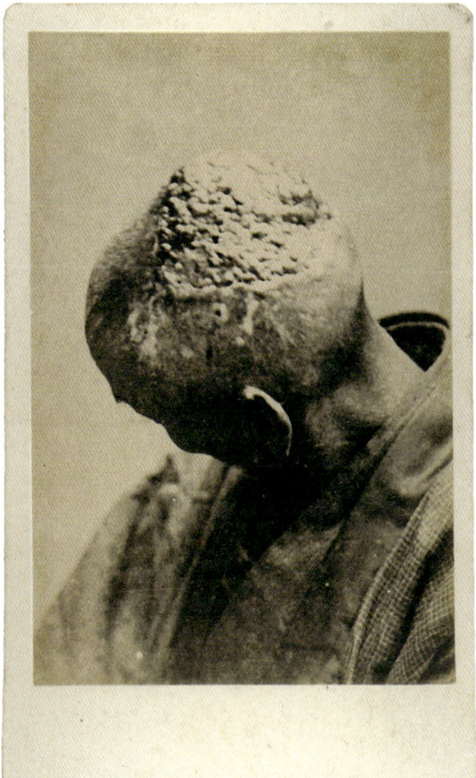

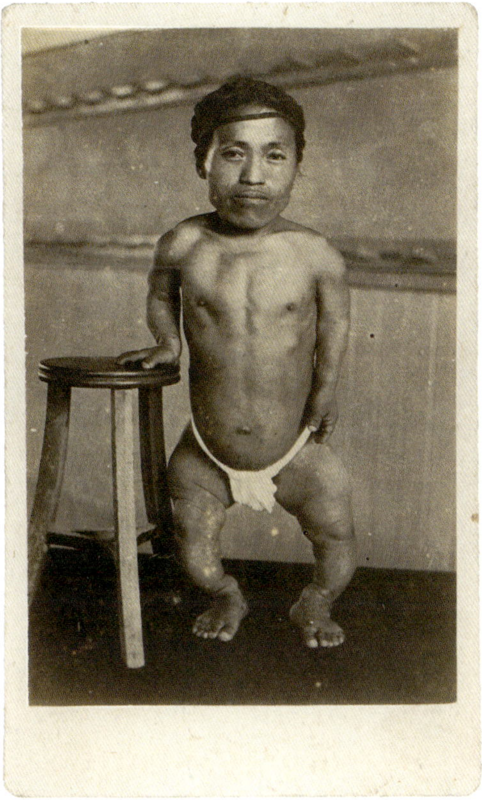

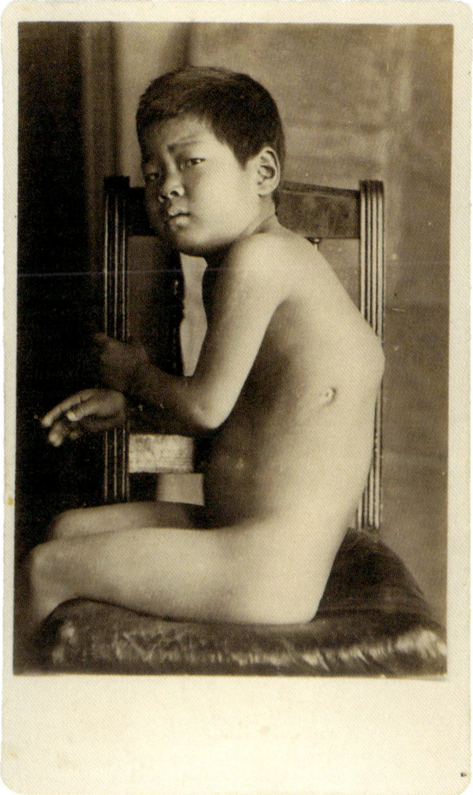

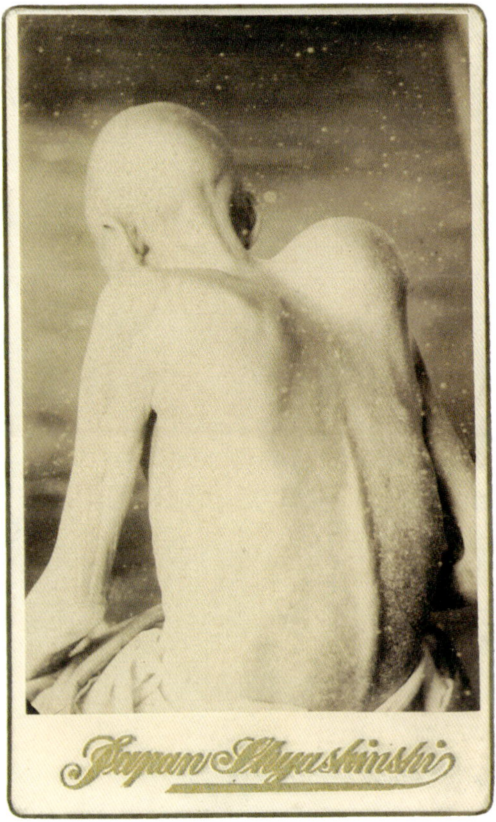

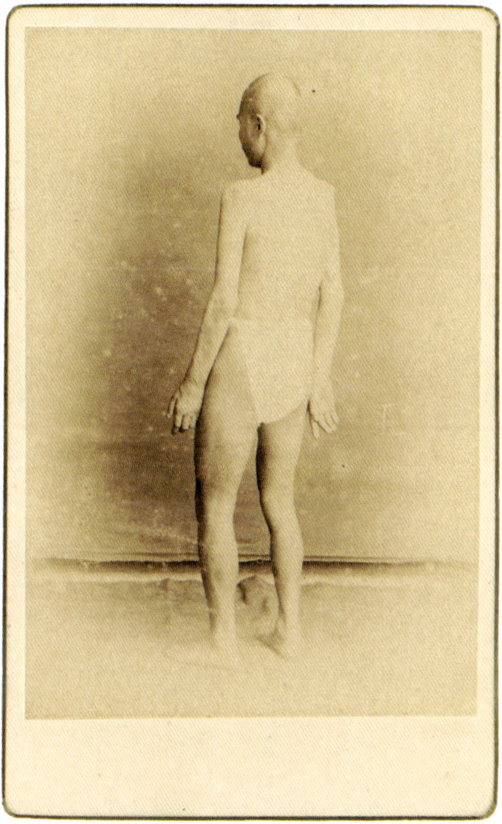

THE HISTORICAL VALUE of this collection of medical photographs is extraordinary. The sheer number of these medical photographs from a medical faculty affiliated with a hospital in the provinces at the end of the 19th century (around 1895) is astounding, as is the fact that they were taken by a professional photographer and have survived to this day. The Kakomachi neighborhood in Hiroshima, where Ochi's practice for internal medicine was located, was in closest proximity to the epicenter of the nuclear bomb dropped by the Americans in World War II. Everything was destroyed there and countless human lives annihilated. If you also take into account that a large part of the other metropolitan areas in Japan went up in flames during the American bombardments, it is almost a miracle that this collection of photographs has survived in such good condition. The decision of the current owner, Akimitsu Naruyama, not to keep this collection as a private treasure but to publish it fills us with respect. It is important that this medical collection—of which neither the descendants of the photographer nor the previous owners had any knowledge—will be preserved and published.

From the viewpoint of the physician, it is not necessarily the case that the diagnostic terminology used 110 years ago is still understandable. Progress in medicine has transformed the classification of diseases, and for this very reason we are able to make much more precise diagnoses. However, many diagnostic terms written on the photographs have remained unchanged. One understands which diseases the physicians of the time were most interested in.

Most of the diseases represented are in an advanced stage (although from a certain point of view you could say this about any disease). They were photographed to document their final phases. The afflicted body parts are all strongly deformed, and you can feel the pain just by looking at the images (the patients themselves naturally experienced strong pains accompanied by fever). The suppuration caused by a swollen stomach or the cyst on an ovary reach proportions hardly ever seen today. There is an astonishing number of malignant tumors, sarcomas for example. Equally astounding is the audacity of the surgical operations at the time—given that anesthesiology was still only very basic. Antibiotics for sterilization and carcinostatic treatments stopping the growth of cancer were still unknown. If the patient was diagnosed with a malignant tumor, he was likely to die shortly after the photosession in most cases.

It seems that there were a lot of patients with malignant tumors in advanced stages—it is astonishing, however, that so few case studies of them were published in medical journals. The massive distension and deformation of organs caused by bacterial infections —nowadays practically unknown thanks to the development of antibiotics—was also photographically documented. A reddening of the epidermis is naturally a fever symptom and seems painful if you just look at the images. Besides bacterial infections, we encounter exemplary images of other diseases extinct today: leprosy, small pox, and many more.

The lay person will notice the genuinely repulsive images of deformed embryos and newborns with anomalies—one-eyed babies, Siamese twins, mutilations, hydrocephali. Collecting rare deformations at European medical faculties has been part of medicine's progress since the Renaissance. Even today preparations of deformed newborns form the core of the most famous anatomical collections in Europe, for example at the universities of Leyden (Netherlands), Montpellier (France), or Riga (Latvia). Although much later, the physicians of Okayama seem to have been guided by a similar interest.

In addition, the photographs show numerous patients with a destroyed nose structure. It remains unclear whether these are injuries due to external influences, or whether these are symptoms of disease. Reconstructive plastic surgery was often performed on these patients. It would be interesting to know where they took the tissue from for this purpose, what type of surgical operation was performed, whether the transplanted tissue died, or whether the transplantation was a lasting success.

The standard of the medical faculty of Okayama and its affiliate hospital was the highest in all of southwestern Japan at that time (around 1895) and was important as a regional center. But the fact that these documentary photographs of over 300 patients have survived in such excellent condition and are now published in book form is not just of great importance to medical historians but also to physicians at large and to the general public.

Sumio Ishida

Senior lecturer for medical history at the medical faculty of the University of Okayama; Member of the board of the Japanese Society for Medical History; Professor at Niimi College

DER HISTORISCHE WERT dieser Sammlung medizinischer Fotografien ist außerordentlich. Die bloße Anzahl dieser medizinischen Aufnahmen von einem an eine Medizinschule angegliederten Spital in der Provinz Ende des 19. Jahrhunderts (um 1895) ist erstaunlich; ebenso die Tatsache, daß sie von einem Fotografen angefertigt wurden und bis heute erhalten geblieben sind. Das Viertel Kakomachi in Hiroshima, wo Ochis Praxis für innere Medizin lag, befindet sich in nächster Nähe zum Epizentrum des Atombombenabwurfs durch die Amerikaner während des Zweiten Weltkriegs. Es wurde dort alles – auch unzählige Menschenleben – vernichtet. Wenn man noch bedenkt, daß die Mehrzahl der japanischen Großstädte während des Zweiten Weltkriegs durch die amerikanischen Bombardierungen in den Flammen untergegangen ist, so grenzt es an ein Wunder, daß diese Fotosammlung bis heute in diesem Zustand erhalten geblieben ist. Daß zudem der gegenwärtige Besitzer, Herr Akimitsu Naruyama, die Sammlung nicht etwa als privaten Schatz hütete, sondern es verstand, sie in dieser Form zu veröffentlichen, erfüllt uns mit Respekt. Es ist wichtig, daß diese medizinische Fotosammlung, von der weder die Nachfahren des Fotografen noch die der früheren Besitzer etwas geahnt hatten, erhalten und publiziert wird.

Es ist keineswegs so, daß die diagnostischen Begriffe, die vor 110 Jahren angewandt wurden, heute für den Mediziner alle verständlich wären. Der Fortschritt in der Medizin veränderte die Klassifizierung der Krankheiten, und so können heute weit präzisere Diagnosen gestellt werden. Viele der auf die Fotografien geschriebenen diagnostischen Begriffe sind jedoch unverändert geblieben. Man versteht, für welche Krankheiten sich die Ärzte damals wirklich interessierten.

Die meisten der abgebildeten Krankheiten sind (auch wenn dies in gewissem Sinn auf jede Krankheit zutrifft) weit fortgeschritten, und sie wurden zur Dokumentation ihres Endstadiums aufgenommen. Die betroffenen Körperteile sind stark deformiert, und man kann den Schmerz beim bloßen Betrachten der Bilder nachempfinden (die Patienten hatten natürlich starke Schmerzen, die von Fieber begleitet wurden). Der Eiterfluß, der eine Bauchschwellung verursacht, und die Zyste am Eierstock erreichen Ausmaße, wie man sie in der Gegenwart kaum mehr sieht. Erstaunlich ist auch die große Anzahl bösartiger Tumore (Krebs), Sarkome und andere. Genauso erstaunt es, welch kühne chirurgische Eingriffe vorgenommen wurden – damals, als nur in Ansätzen Narkosetechnik zur Verfügung stand und weder Antibiotika zur Sterilisierung noch karzinostatische Mittel bekannt waren, die die Ausbreitung bösartiger Tumore hätten verhindern können. Lautete die Diagnose damals auf einen bösartigen Tumor, so ist der Patient in den meisten Fällen wohl kurz nach der Fotoaufnahme gestorben.

Scheinbar gab es damals viele Patienten mit weit fortgeschrittenen, bösartigen Tumoren – erstaunlich ist nur, daß in medizinischen Fachzeitschriften kaum Fallstudien dazu publiziert wurden. Das massive Anschwellen und die Deformation von Organen durch bakterielle Infektionskrankheiten, die heute aufgrund der Entwicklung von Antibiotika beinahe unbekannt sind, wurden ebenfalls fotografisch dokumentiert. Die Rötung der Epidermis ist von Fieber begleitet und wirkt allein beim Betrachten der Bilder sehr schmerzhaft. Nebst bakteriellen Infektionen finden wir auch beispielhafte Aufnahmen von anderen Krankheiten, die heute beinahe ausgestorben sind: Lepra, Pocken und viele weitere.

Dem Laien werden auch die wirklich abstoßenden Bilder mißgebildeter Embryonen und Neugeborener mit Anomalien auffallen, darunter Einäugige, Siamesische Zwillinge, Verstümmelte, Wasserköpfe. Das Sammeln solcher seltener Mißbildungen in Präparatsammlungen gehörte zu den Fortschritten der Schulung an den europäischen Medizinhochschulen seit der Renaissance. Noch heute bilden in den berühmtesten anatomischen Sammlungen Europas – wie beispielsweise an den Universitäten Leiden (Holland), Montpellier (Frankreich) oder Riga (Litauen) – Präparate solcher mißgebildeter Neugeborener den Kern der anatomischen Sammlung. Die Mediziner von Okayama dürften immer noch von einem ähnlichen Interesse geleitet worden sein.

Die Fotografien zeigen auch zahlreiche Patienten mit zerstörter Nasenstruktur, wobei unklar bleibt, ob dies auf äußere Einwirkung oder auf Krankheit zurückführen. Bei diesen Patienten wurden häufig plastische Eingriffe zur Wiederherstellung der Nasenstruktur durchgeführt. Interessant zu wissen wäre, wo dazu Gewebe entnommen, und welche Art von Operation durchgeführt wurde; ob das verpflanzte Gewebe abstarb und von welcher Dauerhaftigkeit die Transplantation war.

Das medizinische Niveau der Medizinhochschule Okayama und des angegliederten Spitals war damals (um 1895) das höchste in Südwestjapan. Daß aber die dokumentarischen Fotografien von über 300 Patienten, die dort in Behandlung waren, in einem so guten Zustand bis heute erhalten geblieben sind und jetzt veröffentlicht werden, ist nicht nur für uns Medizinhistoriker, sondern auch für alle Ärzte und Kliniker, aber auch für das breite Publikum von großer Bedeutung.

Sumio Ishida

Außerordentlicher Lehrbeauftragter für Medizingeschichte an der Medizinischen Fakultät der Universität Okayama; Vorstandsmitglied der Japan Society of Medical History; Lehrbeauftragter am Niimi College

DR. IKKAKU OCHI COLLECTION

Book design: Steidl Design/Claas Möller
Color separations: Steidl Digital Darkroom, Göttingen
Printing and production: Steidl, Göttingen

Head Office: Schifflände 32, CH-8001 Zurich
Switzerland, P.O.Box 73, CH-8024 Zurich/Switzerland
phone: 41 1 261 0910, fax: 41 1 261 9262,
e-mail: publishers@scalo.com, website: www.scalo.com

Distributed in North America by DAP, New York City;
in Europe, Africa, and Asia by Thames and Hudson, London;
in Germany, Austria, and Switzerland by Scalo.

ISBN 3-908247-71-3
Printed in Germany